Body Reshaping through Muscle and Skin Meridian Therapy

An Introduction to 6 Body Types

Body Reshaping through Muscle and Skin Meridian Therapy

An Introduction to 6 Body Types

Jeonhee Jang

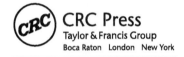

CRC Press
Taylor & Francis Group
Boca Raton London New York

CRC Press is an imprint of the
Taylor & Francis Group, an **informa** business

CRC Press
Taylor & Francis Group
6000 Broken Sound Parkway NW, Suite 300
Boca Raton, FL 33487-2742

© 2016 by Taylor & Francis Group, LLC
CRC Press is an imprint of Taylor & Francis Group, an Informa business

No claim to original U.S. Government works

Printed on acid-free paper
Version Date: 20151207

International Standard Book Number-13: 978-1-4987-5873-4 (Hardback)

This book contains information obtained from authentic and highly regarded sources. Reasonable efforts have been made to publish reliable data and information, but the author and publisher cannot assume responsibility for the validity of all materials or the consequences of their use. The authors and publishers have attempted to trace the copyright holders of all material reproduced in this publication and apologize to copyright holders if permission to publish in this form has not been obtained. If any copyright material has not been acknowledged please write and let us know so we may rectify in any future reprint.

Except as permitted under U.S. Copyright Law, no part of this book may be reprinted, reproduced, transmitted, or utilized in any form by any electronic, mechanical, or other means, now known or hereafter invented, including photocopying, microfilming, and recording, or in any information storage or retrieval system, without written permission from the publishers.

For permission to photocopy or use material electronically from this work, please access www.copyright.com (http://www.copyright.com/) or contact the Copyright Clearance Center, Inc. (CCC), 222 Rosewood Drive, Danvers, MA 01923, 978-750-8400. CCC is a not-for-profit organization that provides licenses and registration for a variety of users. For organizations that have been granted a photocopy license by the CCC, a separate system of payment has been arranged.

Trademark Notice: Product or corporate names may be trademarks or registered trademarks, and are used only for identification and explanation without intent to infringe.

Library of Congress Cataloging-in-Publication Data

Names: Jang, Jeonhee, author.
Title: Body reshaping through muscle and skin meridian therapy : an introduction to 6 body types / Jeonhee Jang.
Description: Boca Raton : Taylor & Francis, 2015. | Includes index.
Identifiers: LCCN 2015047410 | ISBN 9781498758734 (alk. paper)
Subjects: | MESH: Musculoskeletal Manipulations--methods | Meridians | Body Image
Classification: LCC QP301 | NLM WB 535 | DDC 612.7--dc23
LC record available at http://lccn.loc.gov/2015047410

Visit the Taylor & Francis Web site at
http://www.taylorandfrancis.com

and the CRC Press Web site at
http://www.crcpress.com

Contents

Author xiii

Chapter 1 Body Reshaping for Health and Beauty.................................... 1

Perfect 10.. 1
Learning from Man's Best Friend.. 2
Balancing and Reshaping Your Body 3
Body Posture 4
Having a Healthy Body Shape 4
Beauty Is Not Only Skin Deep 6
Skin and Thermoregulation 7
Subcutaneous Fat.. 8
Food, Fitness, and Fat 10
Resetting Your Digestive System 11
And You Thought Losing Weight Was Simple?............................... 12

Chapter 2 A First Look at the Meridian System in TCM................... 13

Understanding the Essentials (Qi and Meridian) 13
Obesity Is Developed Step by Step 14
Spleen Functions in TCM.. 14
Autonomic Nervous System and Spleen Function..................... 14
Transportation and Transformation of Spleen Function in TCM........ 15
Dampness in Spleen Function Imbalance in TCM..................... 15
Extremities and Muscle: Spleen Function in TCM.................... 15
Diaphragm and Congestion in Abdominal Cavity.................... 16
Body Cavities and Body Fluids... 16
Dampness, Edema, and Disorders 17
San Jiao (Triple Burner) in TCM and Body Cavities 17
Healthy Habits and Circadian Rhythm 18
Circadian Rhythms and the Meridian Clock.................................. 19
Sleep and Wakefulness: Homeostatic Balance 20
Parallels between Asian and Western Medicine.............................. 20

Chapter 3 Who Can Benefit from This Treatment? 21

Weight Loss or Diet Life versus My Life... 21
Body Reshaping and Successful Health Regimens 22
Subcutaneous Fat.. 23
Postchildbirth Complications.. 24

v

vi • *Contents*

Caesarean Section..24
Adhesion-Related Disorder 25
Functional Gastrointestinal Disorders 26
Major Scars 27
   Types of Scar..27
   Stretch Marks...28
Cellulite..28
Peripheral Neuropathies...28
Emotional Expression by the Body 29
TMJ...30
Bruxism..32
Depression and Anxiety 32
Medication History Complications: Allergy Medication 33
Obesity 33

Chapter 4   Body Posture and Homeostasis....................................35

Chinese Medicine, Balance, and Homeostasis..............................36
Wu Xing...37
TCM Life Cycles 37
   Biological Rhythms 38
   Kidney and Kidney Essence 38
Eight Principles: Pattern of Body Balance Identification................39
   Exterior versus Interior Identification 39
   Hot and Cold Identifications...40
   Vacuity (Deficiency) and Repletion (Excess) Identification 40
   Yin and Yang Identification...40
Homeostasis 40
   Water and Salt Intake and Body Fluid Homeostasis 41
Immune Function and Thermoregulation......................................43
   Respiratory System and Homeostasis 44
   Blood pH Homeostasis...45
   Bone (Calcium and Phosphate) Homeostasis 47
Understanding Body Homeostasis and Metabolism........................47
   Lifestyle and Homeostasis 49
   Understanding Structure versus Function..............................50
Eight Extraordinary Meridians 51
   Du Channel..52
   Ren Channel 52
   Chong Channel 52
   Dai Channel...54
   Yang and Yin Heel Channels...54
Yang and Yin Linking Channels..55

Contents • vii

Chapter 5 Six Body Types 59

Purpose of Differentiation.. 59
Background 59
Treat Branches and Root 60
Criteria of the Six Body Types 60
Characteristics of the Six Body Types 61
Type P 62
    Quick Tips.. 62
    Related Conditions 62
    Clinical Syndrome 63
        Body Trunk Pressed and Extremities Depressed 63
        Body Trunk Depressed and Extremities Pressed 63
        Skin Tension—Muscle Weak 64
        Skin Weak—Muscle Tension 64
    Understanding the Mechanism 65
        Skeletal Muscles.. 65
        Blood Vessels in Skin and Skeletal Muscle 66
        Breathing and Circulation = Air and Food............................ 66
    Pain 66
    Postural Characteristics.. 67
    Possible Associated Disorders 67
    Treatment... 67
    Simple Home Therapy and Caution 68
    Case Study.. 68
        Brief History 68
        Observations... 69
        Assessments and Plan... 69
Type T... 70
    Quick Tips.. 70
    Related Conditions 70
    Clinical Syndrome 71
    Understanding the Mechanism 72
        Immune System Lymph 72
        Transportation of Nutrient: Lymph System........................... 72
        Lymph Fluid Accumulation 73
        Venous Insufficiency... 73
        Gaining Weight 73
    Pain 74
    Postural Characteristics.. 75
    Possible Associated Disorders 75
    Treatment... 75
        Simple Home Care and Cautions.. 76

viii • *Contents*

Case Study 76
    Brief History 77
    Observations 77
Type S 78
  Quick Tips 78
  Related Conditions 78
  Clinical Syndrome 79
  Chong and Yin Wei Type (Heart and Digestive System) 79
    Characteristics 79
  Dai and Yang Wei Type (Liver and Immune System) 80
    Characteristics 80
  Ren and Yin Qiao Type (Lung and Circulatory System) 80
    Characteristics 80
  Du and Yang Qiao Type (Kidney and Nervous System) 81
    Characteristics 81
  Understanding the Mechanism 82
    Lipedema 82
  Pain 83
    Mechanical Joint Pain 83
    Metabolic Joint Pain 84
  Postural Characteristics 84
    Possible Associated Disorders 84
    Treatment 84
    Simple Home Therapy and Caution 85
  Case Study 85
    Brief History 85
    Observations 86
    Treatment Plan and Assessment 86

Chapter 6   Anatomical Approach: Types M1, M2, and M3 89

Type M1 89
  Quick Tips 89
  Related Condition 89
  Clinical Syndrome 90
  Understanding the Mechanism 90
    Pain 92
    Muscle Connection and Function in Type M1 93
    Postural Characteristics 93
    Possible Associated Disorders 94
    Simple Home Therapy and Caution 94
  Case Study 94
    Brief History 94

Observations 95
Assessment and Plan (Treatment Plan) 96
Results 97
Type M2 98
Quick Tips 98
Related Condition 99
Clinical Syndrome 99
Understanding the Mechanism 100
Type M2 Muscle Connections and Functions 101
Pain 103
Postural Characteristics 104
Possible Associated Disorders 104
Treatment 104
Simple Home Care and Cautions 105
Case Study 106
Brief History 106
Observations 106
Assessment and Plan 107
Type M3 107
Quick Tips 107
Related Condition 108
Clinical Syndrome 108
Understanding the Mechanism 110
Body Balance 110
Muscle Sequential Connection and Function for Type M3 111
Type M3 and Blood Circulation 112
Pain 113
Postural Characteristics 114
Possible Associated Disorders 114
Treatment 114
Simple Home Therapy and Precautions 115
Case Study 116
Observations 116
Brief History 116
Assessment and Treatment 117

Chapter 7 Muscle Meridian Therapy and Skin Cutaneous Therapy 121

What are Muscle and Sinew Meridians and Cutaneous Meridians? 121
Classification of Connective Tissues 122
Meridian Classifications 122
Six Body Types and Muscle Meridians 122
Muscle Meridian Treatments for Six Body Type Groups 123

_x_ • _Contents_

Characteristics of Muscle Meridians 124
    Nourish the Muscles, Tendons, and Skin 124
    Three Yang and Three Yin Hand and Foot Meridians 125
    Muscle Meridian Pathogenic Patterns 125
    Muscle Meridians Originate from Distal Body Parts 126
Muscle Meridian 126
Three Hand Yang Meridians 127
    Hand Tai Yang Small Intestine Meridian Flow 127
    Hand Shao Yang San Jiao (Triple Burner) Meridian Flow 127
    Hand Yang Ming Large Intestine Meridian Flow 128
Three Hand Yin Meridians 128
    Hand Tai Yin Lung Muscle Meridian Flow 129
    Hand Jue Yin Pericardium Muscle Meridian Flow 129
    Hand Shao Yin Heart Meridian Flow 130
    Hand Yin Muscle Meridian Reference 130
Three Foot Yang Meridians 132
    Clinical Syndrome 132
    Foot Tai Yang Urinary Bladder Meridian Flow 132
    Foot Shao Yang Gallbladder Meridian Flow 133
    Foot Yang Ming Stomach Meridian Flow 133
Three Foot Yin Meridians 134
    Clinical Syndrome 134
    Foot Tai Yin Spleen Muscle Meridian Flow 134
    Foot Jue Yin Liver Meridian Flow 135
    Foot Shao Yin Kidney Meridian Flow 135

Cutaneous Meridian 136
    Function of Skin 137
    Six Body Types and Skin 137
        Diagnosis for the Skin Meridian 137
        Treatment of the Skin Meridian 138
        Clinical Syndrome 138
        Tai Yang Cutaneous Meridian Pattern 138
        Shao Yang Cutaneous Meridian Pattern 139
        Yang Ming Cutaneous Meridian Pattern 139
        Tai Yin Cutaneous Meridian Pattern 140
        Jue Yin Cutaneous Meridian Pattern 140
        Shao Yin Cutaneous Meridian Pattern 141
    Myotome and Dermatome 141

Chapter 8 Treatment Methods 143

Clinical Setting 143
    Muscle Meridian Acupuncture Technique 143
        Summary of the Muscle Meridian Technique 144

Contents • xi

Cupping...144
   Contraindications of Cupping Therapy.............................144
Moxa Oil and Gua Sha...145
Hyperthermal Methods 146
   Moxibustion...146
   Ja-Hun...147
Gastrointestinal Resuscitation 147
   Benefits of GIR...148
CPR versus GIR..148
Acupressure 148
   Characteristics of Acupressure Therapy............................148
Home Setting...149
Half-Body Bath...149
   Benefits of Herbal Bath Treatments.................................150
   Scrub and Moxa Soap..150
Muscle Meridian Stretching...150
   Connect Your Inner Motions...150
   Practice Moving Your Hands and Feet Slowly and Gently...151
   Circular Motions...151
Diet and Nutrition 152
   Diet Recommendations..152
   Sleep and Breakfast Habit 152
Personal Planning...153

Chapter 9 Specific Clinical Cautions and Application 155

Muscle Meridian Acupuncture Needling 155
Needle Pinpoint Allergic Reaction...155
Sore Muscles and a Heavy Feeling after Needling 155
Bruising..155
Tiredness, Fatigue, and Sleep 156
Gastrointestinal Resuscitation and Moxa Treatment.............................156
Loose Stool and Gurgling Sound..156
Hypochondriac Itchiness..156
Bloating and Nausea...156
Moxa Oil and Gua Sha...156
Bruising..156
Allergic Reaction..157
Cupping...157
Petechia 157

Appendix: Facial Rejuvenation from Asian Wisdom.................................159

Index...163

Author

Jeonhee Jang has more than 20 years of comprehensive exposure to both Eastern and Western medicine, through both her formal and extensive education and her earlier experience working with her mother, who is a Moxibustion specialist in Korea.

Jeonhee earned a master of science degree in Oriental medicine from the Acupuncture and Integrative Medicine College in Berkeley, California, and a master of education degree from Boston University, Boston, Massachusetts, where she majored in health education focused on the prevention of STDs and AIDS.

Jeonhee earned a bachelor's degree from Ewha Womans University in Seoul, Korea, where she majored in health education, and earned her high school teaching license for military nursing education.

Today Jeonhee works at her acupuncture clinic and wellness center in San Francisco, where she helps her patients with integrated assessment and treatment from both Eastern and Western medicine.

1

Body Reshaping for Health and Beauty

PERFECT 10

Today, many people take for granted that our primary standard for beauty is based on how closely we can synchronize our bodies with images from the commercial worlds of advertising or celebrity. Yet, a little-appreciated fact is that we also equate such images with health. What results from the combined effects of false body shape and misconceptions about what is healthy is an overload of information, or indeed misinformation, about not only how to achieve the desired body shape, but also how our health and lifestyles are dictated by it.

Once someone has achieved perceived "good results" from such information or therapies, then understandably enough, he or she wants to share his or her news with others. Social media networks and private blogs have contributed greatly to spreading these experiences and results, many of which are supported by photos or video clips that seek to substantiate the claims. There is no denying that much good can be spread by social media, and indeed, there are many advantages, particularly with respect to informing others about sources derived from cultures worldwide, but all this can result in "too much of a good thing."

Information overload, and particularly that which is spread at lightning speed by the Internet, can result in a bias with harmful negative effects. Rarely do people question the information; they simply follow the instructions without considering that their own condition not only might fail to improve, but also could be made even worse. The result, then, may be not only a negative social effect, but also a negative health effect.

Another issue that arises relative to a picture-perfect reflection of other people's body shape and looks, especially in adolescent groups, is how they can develop their own false body image from those of celebrities or models. Models, in particular, have body shapes that sometimes border on the extraordinary because these shapes are essentially manufactured and manipulated simply to make the clothes they wear look better. In this case, designers indirectly dictate the health status of adolescents.

1

For males, the heavily muscled, tanned stereotype trends strongly reflect not only a body image, but also how a healthy young man should look. Even in adult males, this perception predominates and gyms are full of men trying to achieve this aim. In the case of young females, even in cultures where the curvy figure was once valued, they now aspire to the thinner models they see on catwalks and in the pages of their favorite magazines.

Yet, despite negative effects on health, the influence of such role models is stronger now than it ever has been. This is because, subconsciously, we mimic the looks and behavior of people we like—an effect known as mirroring in psychology. This effect is now considered to be even stronger in regard to those outside our network of personal acquaintances, simply because we spend more time looking at such images in magazines, on TV, or on a computer screen than we do in face-to-face situations. This fact is probably obvious if you consider how easily a new fashion or hairstyle is soon copied by almost every young person you know or see in the street.

We are not, of course, images; neither are we photoshopped on the pages of a magazine or on a website. We are real people who react when touched and our skin feels nothing like the pages of a glossy magazine or a computer monitor.

To change our concept of who we are, we first have to accept that we are not the same person as the image we covet. Even if we wear the same clothes, cosmetics, or hairstyle, chances are we will still look completely different. The toned bodies and glistening abdominal muscles of the people we admire do not belong to us, if, considering digital manipulation, they exist in reality at all.

LEARNING FROM MAN'S BEST FRIEND

We all have different attractions and, when discussing body image and health with my clients, I usually explain the differences between who and what we are as individuals by looking at my favorite pet, the dog. Dog breeds are all different with regard to both body shape and character. Greyhounds, for example, have a lean shape with long legs. The dachshund has a long waist and short legs. Poodles have curly hair and a small face, and the bulldog has a big face and wide shoulders. Yet, people consider not only particular dog breeds as gorgeous, but also those of mixed lineage. We do not want all dogs to look and behave alike. Indeed, it would seem strange if we did. However, dogs prove to us that there is much truth in the old adage "beauty is in the eye of the beholder," because we are all, in our own way, beautiful enough not only to be loved, but also to love ourselves.

Yet our attraction to the different breeds of dogs also identifies another contradiction between how we view ourselves and how we view our pets. If our pets are sick, we notice. We are immediately aware of their ailments through observing not only their physical state, but also their behavior. If these factors change in some way, for example, with regard to eating, sleeping, walking, running, barking, a change in body shape, or unexplained inactivity, then we immediately notice. We notice, too, if they show sudden weight gain, develop a depression in the spine, start to itch, or have abdominal bloating, an unusual gait, or irregular breathing. We know when they are in a healthy condition, and therefore we recognize when they are ill or functioning at less than their optimal level. We notice, too, when their health is restored and they are back to normal. Yet rarely we give ourselves the same consideration.

What we can learn from our own behavior toward the dog is that it is not how we look and behave compared to others that counts. What does count is that personal status in terms of health and beauty is of far more importance, and we need to balance ourselves physically, emotionally, and environmentally.

Our definition of beauty needs redefining because what it really should be is a quality or a combination of qualities that gives pleasure to the mind or senses, rather than being something we appreciate only visually. Beauty is *you* and should incorporate harmony of form, color, proportion, authenticity, and of course, originality.

BALANCING AND RESHAPING YOUR BODY

It is so important that we change our perception of what health actually means. Being healthy does not simply mean we are free from medical intervention or treatment, but that we have the ability to adapt our own health status. This means we also have to look at background, lifestyle, economic and social conditions, and individual spirituality. Balancing and reshaping the body are only the first steps toward designing a different and better lifestyle and finding your own way to be whom you truly want to be.

Once you have accepted that your own beauty is not simply a desired image based on that of someone else, you can start to balance and reshape your own body. I cannot stress strongly enough that this is not to achieve a "fashionable shape," but to maximize your own health. When you are healthy, your natural and most attractive shape will automatically follow—the shape that suits *you*.

Many people view the issues associated with body shape as being something distinctive from their health. When it comes to weight, they think of it in terms of fat, calories, dieting, and exercise. In this book, I show you how your weight and body shape can be a direct result of ill health, and the structures and functions that are involved. We explore much more than just what your scale and the fit of your clothes might tell you; in this book, we look at

- Skin
- Fat
- Muscles
- Diaphragm
- Historical illness or injuries
- Body posture
- Body clock or circadian rhythm
- Digestion
- Blood vessels
- Nutrition
- Sympathetic nervous system
- Parasympathetic nervous system
- Enteric nervous system

By examining the above factors, you will learn how they contribute toward changes in body shape. Nowhere, you might note, have I mentioned either dieting or exercise.

The starting point in this process is to create your own simple journal to establish your current health status and possibly reveal how you came to reach this point. This is not a complicated or detailed task; simply make a timeline of any events directly related to health problems, for example, 1999 C-section or 2000 chiropractic treatment for lower back pain. It is also essential to include personal observations, for example, "2004 enrolled college, sitting all day, back pain started" or "2006 weight below 119 pounds due *to* playing tennis and swimming."

Looking back over these events will assist you and your practitioner in establishing whether there is a connection between your current health status and past events. Many people fail to make these connections simply because they feel they are too busy to do it or are afraid of the worst-case scenario. However, in order to resolve your current health issues, it is essential that you examine the past and thus ensure that you can learn from it as necessary with the help of your practitioner.

BODY POSTURE

The next task is to examine your own body posture, and the best way to do this is to ask someone to take photos of you while you are sitting, standing, and walking. You will be able to clearly see any obvious postural issues. You can also take note of the postural position you find most comfortable. This might be sitting at your work desk, watching TV, or standing.

Next, you need to think about restriction of movement. Do you notice that your ankles or neck only have limited rotation? Is it difficult for you to bend, either forward or to the side? When you have established that an area has restricted movement, palpate it with your fingers to see if you can feel any abnormalities. These may be due to slight swellings, stringy sections, or a hardening underneath the skin surface. Any abnormalities such as these do not mean you have a disease, but they can be potential health problems and ultimately result in chronic illnesses.

For example, the lower back area may feel cold and a "watery" lump may be apparent at each side. It may also show an abnormal stretch mark that is a little lighter in color. This is not just a simple fat deposit. It can cause lower back pain, sleep disorders, or digestion issues, particularly problems with bowel movements. It can also cause a lipoma to form, which is a noncancerous deposit of fatty cells.

As another example, you follow the Achilles tendon area on each side and discover a swelling on one side. If the swelling is on the inside, this can be because of circulation problems, while a swelling on the outer side can be due to misalignment of the pelvis and hip.

Although this form of self-examination may seem a little unusual, it is no different from that of the breast self-examination that doctors recommend women perform on themselves.

HAVING A HEALTHY BODY SHAPE

It should seem quite natural that good health comes from having the right body position and posture. When I talk of a good body shape, what I really mean is that you have a good body posture. Maintaining an optimal body position means that it is aligned, requires the least muscle involvement to maintain, and places the least strain on ligaments and bones as they fight gravity.

Good posture is not limited to walking around; it is required when sitting, standing, and moving. When taking part in sporting activities, posture is of prime consideration to prevent adverse effects arising from structural problems. As athletes know, not only do injuries result from poor posture as relevant to their particular sport, but good posture results in better performance.

Maintaining a particular posture puts stress on various parts of the body and in particular muscles, which results in continuous low-level contraction. When our muscles contract, our nervous system makes adjustments by contracting blood vessels and adjusting oxygen levels within different sections of the body. This physiologic mechanism consumes energy, and all this has to be done by the body against the effects of gravity. Only during deep sleep do our muscles escape the pull of gravity. And it is only during the rapid eye movement (REM) sleep phase that our skeletal muscles are paralyzed, except, of course, those of the autonomous muscles that keep us alive, such as the diaphragm. The paralysis of skeletal muscles during this part of our sleep pattern is one reason why we can never go into a deep sleep when standing up.

We may believe that muscles and bones are only required for movement, but in reality they are only the structural part of the operation. Blood vessels and the nervous system, the respiratory system, the abdominal activity regulated by the digestive system, and many other systemic functions are all involved, and each function can affect the maintenance of our posture.

In my personal clinical observations, I see muscular imbalance arising from habit, trauma, genetics, and repetitive use, resulting in local "congestion," the excessive accumulation of a body fluid or pain. Localized congestion can become chronic and subsequently influence the range of motion or result in a permanent change of posture. Body pain from skeletal imbalance results in immobility and thus can result in muscle dystrophy, which is a progressive weakening of the muscles resulting in loss of muscle mass, and which can permanently limit range of motion and cause postural change. For example, if we are injured in any way and alter our movement because of it, muscle weakness may start to develop in the area we are not using. It then becomes a habit, leading to permanent atrophy of the muscle group concerned even though the original injury, for instance, a broken bone, has long since been repaired.

Muscle imbalances occur when certain muscles become short and tight, while the antagonist (opposite muscles) often become long and weak. The shortened and tightened muscles are usually postural muscles and, as the name suggests, are those involved in maintaining our posture. The lengthened and weakened muscles are those involved in movement, which are known as the phasic muscles. Both muscle types are renowned for responding in this manner to poor posture and injury.

If we have poor posture, our body needs to work harder against gravity to maintain the position, which then leads to fatigue and tiredness. It also creates a heavier load on ligaments, which in turn can lead to bone deformity and inflammation. Once this situation occurs, other functions, such as respiration, digestion, or circulation, are all affected, and the resulting tendonitis or arthritis further aggravates the problems.

Although we might believe otherwise, a functional problem in the body affecting its structure, such as a bone fracture, does not affect the body in isolation because the effects are both internal and external. When a bone heals, there is the possibility of some level of deformity that can result in a different postural angle. Although this angle may be very slight, any unusual angular movement puts stress on other muscles and ligaments, and this results in responses that, through the sensation, can develop into back pain, which in turn disturbs the autonomic nervous system that regulates our internal organ systems.

In my clinic, I saw many examples of this while treating patients. Unlike the thoracic spine, the neck and lower back area connect with both the cervical and pelvic bones that move side by side and up and down. These movements need the flexibility of the surrounding muscles and soft tissue. If these areas are tight, for example, when the neck is rigid due to a car accident, then the body is not in parasympathetic mode. The pelvis and head are connected by the spine area, which must be flexible and soft to allow for circular movements. This is similar to the hula dance you can perform in certain important areas, like the neck, hip, wrist, and ankle.

BEAUTY IS NOT ONLY SKIN DEEP

The skin is a symbol of beauty as well as the manifestation of body healthy condition. It is the largest organ of the body and has many functions, including physical and mechanical protection, thermoregulation, immunologic action, and sensation. The outermost layer of the skin is called the epidermis, and not only does it provide a protective role, but it also regulates water loss, which prevents internal organs from drying out. The skin also provides a physical barrier against exterior pathogenic factors such as sunlight, viruses, bacteria, and

harmful chemicals. Since the skin has this important barrier role, it connects to the central nervous system, which works with the peripheral nervous system. This means that it sends signals from the periphery, or outside, through the dermis, subcutaneous fat, and epidermis, back to our spinal cord and onto the brain.

The nerve networks of the skin contain somatic sensory and sympathetic autonomic fibers. The sensory nerves function as receptors of touch, pain, temperature, itch, and mechanical stimuli. Distribution of these nerve functions is not standard, but varies across the skin's surface, with the denser areas of nerve endings usually found on hairless parts of the body. Sympathetic motor fibers run with the sensory nerves in the dermis until they branch off to innervate the sweat glands, vascular smooth muscles, arrector pili muscles of hair follicles, and sebaceous glands.

Under normal circumstances, the skin is involved with the sympathetic nervous system in that it responds to external stimuli. The skin is governed by not only nerves, but also peripheral blood, lymphatic fluids, and its own personal army of defense, the white blood cells. Many people participate in certain activities to increase the flow of such fluids and cells to bring them to the surface of the skin and so increase their effectiveness. However, if you put the skin and the systems supporting it under extreme pressure, for example, such as that associated with using a sauna or being exposed to extreme cold, then the skin itself becomes traumatized as blood is redirected.

The skin is like an army in battle; it needs sentries and alarm mechanisms to provide protection from external enemies, and these are provided by the central nervous system. In support of this, the skin depends on the peripheral blood circulation and lymphatic body fluids to provide the nutrients while battling any rogue cells. This process is supported by a further army, that of the white blood cells.

While treating chronic pain patients with conditions such as fibromyalgia, skin treatment can be a very helpful aid to the other core treatments. Patients suffering from depression and stress have better results from entire body skin treatment than other, more local modalities. Cutaneous vasodilation is the key balancing skin treatment, and cupping, gua sha, and moxa treatments can be applied locally or to the entire body. In my clinical treatment protocol, chronic pain patients and those with depression and stress are given these skin relaxation treatments, which bring about benefits for the entire body.

Preventing the signs of early aging means being kind not only to your skin, but also to that which lies beneath it.

The dermis is the inner, thicker layer of skin and provides both flexibility and mechanical strength. An integrated system of connective tissue elements, it also accommodates a network of nerves and blood vessels. Fibroblasts make up the all-important collagen, which tightens the skin. When you are younger, you have an abundance of these cells. However, as you age, they diminish and your skin, as most women are aware, becomes less taut and youthful. Fibroblasts also play a role in promoting interactions between the inner dermis and the outer epidermis.

The skin also contains macrophages, and these address wound healing on the skin, producing what is known as granulation as new skin begins to form, ultimately forming scarring. Mast cells are also regular residents of the dermis and contain not only histamine, which is responsible for allergic

reactions, but also heparin—an anticoagulant that stems bleeding. Heparin also plays an important role in what is known as angiogenesis. This is the process of new blood vessels branching out from preexisting ones; these are essential for promoting healing. This means that mast cells are responsible for the immediate type of hypersensitivity reaction in your skin and are involved in subacute and chronic inflammatory processes.

This protective framework also promotes interactions between the inner dermis and the outer epidermis, in addition to being involved in wound healing and scarring. It may now be the case that there is an information overload regarding collagen synthesis by fibroblasts. For example, blood cells tell scleroderma fibroblasts to produce collagen, and the result is that many patients then suffer from information overload.

More details of this case can be found in Chapter 5, where I look in detail at the different body types and explain the possible long-term effects on other patients in a similar situation.

SKIN AND THERMOREGULATION

When we feel hot, we sweat to keep our body temperature stable. Sweating is a response triggered by the area of the brain where the hypothalamus is located, and acts as the body's thermostat. As the body core temperature rises, the hypothalamus triggers the eccrine glands to produce moisture that emerges on the skin's surface. The eccrine sweat glands are found all over the skin and open directly onto the surface. The highest density is found in the palms of the hands and on the soles of the feet.

Heat is not the only trigger for sweating; other triggers are emotional stress, exercise, hormonal changes, food, disease, and infection. Apocrine glands differ from eccrine glands in several ways, not only in that they are present in certain areas such as the axillae (armpits), areola and nipples of the breast, ear canal, eyelids, nose, and groin area, and usually respond to stress or stimulation. Only the apocrine glands produce the distinctive sweaty odor.

Some people believe that sweating can detoxify the body, and they induce sweating for this reason. However, after sweating, the feeling of being refreshed relates to the volume of lost body fluids rather than getting rid of toxic substances. Most sweat contains water, salt, and some fatty acid and proteins from the apocrine gland. However, if you sweat because of exercise, your body will excrete predominantly salt and water, causing your body to dehydrate.

Skin conditions are important and often provide telltale signs of internal discomfort or disease. An imbalance in factors affecting the homeostasis—the body's ability to maintain a stable internal environment—may manifest as a wrinkle, hair loss, blisters, rashes, and even skin cancer. For example, diabetes manifests itself in a particular skin condition, providing doctors with the ability to better diagnose or sometimes eliminate other illnesses.

Traditional Chinese medicine (TCM) regards the skin as extremely important since signs and symptoms are observed in its patterns, color, texture, turgor, temperature, and quality. Each pattern also corresponds with skin symptoms and signs pertaining to the internal organ symptoms. TCM refers to treating the root, the primary problem, and treating the branch, the secondary problem. This holds particularly true when it comes to the skin. Skin disorder patients can suffer not only physically but also mentally because it affects their appearance.

SUBCUTANEOUS FAT

Subcutaneous fat, which is also known as skin fat, lies directly beneath the skin layers. Looking healthy and younger is related to the distribution of subcutaneous fat, and so some people have fat injections to give them a wrinkle-free, younger-looking face. In this case, fat is taken from another part of the body and injected into the face to smooth out fine lines.

Yet, outside of our own cosmetic interests, subcutaneous fat has several serious duties to perform. It protects the skin, insulates the body, stores energy, and allows for skin mobility with underlying structures. The largest blood vessels of the skin are found in the subcutaneous fat that lies just beneath the skin, and these transport nutrients and circulate immune system cells. The dermis or inner layer of skin and subcutaneous fat are structurally and functionally integrated through a network of nerves and vessels. If there is too little subcutaneous fat, wound healing can be delayed.

Excessive subcutaneous fat accumulation disturbs the hormonal system and limits the range of body motion; yet, reducing subcutaneous fat is achieved far more easily by exercise than is the case with visceral fat. Visceral fat responds more effectively to changes in diet, but excesses are not limited to eating too much or a lack of movement. It is related more to the possibility of chronic inflammation, indigestion, scar tissue adhesion, and a host of other issues. Visceral fat is now linked to the natural immune response system and most of the chronic conditions that afflict many people in modern society.

When I treat patients, I explain that the subcutaneous fat and body shape are related to the distribution of fatty tissue. This, in itself, is influenced by the condition beneath the fat rather than the fat itself. Fat can accumulate in this way because of the condition of muscles or aponeuroses, which are sheets of flat broad tendons. If the condition of muscles and tendons is improved, then the skin surface starts to change and the subcutaneous fat distribution is affected. This is because muscle and skin are connected and move together.

There can be no doubt that exercise not only makes us feel good, but also helps to maintain a good body shape. However, too much exercise results in muscles tightening and the skin becoming thinner. Moreover, excessive exercise causes the skin and muscles to disconnect, resulting in skin feeling looser rather than tighter. If you have lost weight but your abdominal area still has fatty tissue, then that is proof that you are losing the skin fat but still have nonsubcutaneous abdominal fat to lose.

Having abdominal fat is more dependent on your daily habits than on exercise. Sitting is a major contributor to abdominal area congestion because the diaphragm is expanded and abdominal muscles are compressed, allowing the waist circumference to expand. Spinal tension from sitting can result in shallow breathing and sluggish digestion. Skin fat can be controlled by physical activity, but abdominal fat is controlled by the organ systems, especially digestion, breathing, and peripheral circulatory systems.

In my clinical experience, mild skin abnormalities are often related to chronic inflammation from local congestion where localized fluids cause fat to distribute unevenly. Take, for instance, the deposits known as cellulite, with which many women concern themselves. These dimpled areas are rarely related to being overweight specifically. In fact, many underweight women still suffer from cellulite in the same way that overweight women do. Cellulite is usually related to a musculoskeletal problem rather than fat accumulation, particularly on the thighs.

Many women will testify that dieting and exercise have little effect on cellulite, and this is for good reason. To rid yourself of cellulite, you have to look at the underlying cause, which is usually related to the pelvis and legs. Once corrections to muscle and skin in these areas have been effected, the cellulite will start to disappear. If the problem is related to the posture or an internal adhesion, then this will result in uneven subcutaneous fat distribution— which is exactly what cellulite is. The cause of wrinkles or cellulite is not actually linked to problems with the skin but to a postural problem or internal adhesion under the skin. This results in uneven subcutaneous fat distribution and so results in stretch marks, wrinkles, or cellulite. When it comes to such skin problems, the solution is to treat the body directly under the problem area or "on the spot."

Fat should not be considered in isolation. When we consider fat, we have to appreciate that the skin's surface and epidermal appendages (such as glands) are supplied with blood from the dermal vessels from musculocutaneous arteries that penetrate the subcutaneous fat and enter the deep, reticular dermis. In other words, the skin is rooted to muscles and the vessels need to travel from the muscle, through all the different layers, and onto the skin—this is particularly relevant on the trunk and extremities.

A similar situation appears with what are known as epidermal appendages, such as hair follicles, sweat glands, and mammary glands that, although they appear at the surface of the skin, are formed within the body and into the dermis. They, too, are supplied with blood from dermal vessels, which in themselves are branches from musculocutaneous arteries that penetrate the subcutaneous fat.

FOOD, FITNESS, AND FAT

Many in the West have grown accustomed to eating large food portions, whether at home or in restaurants. Yet, in many countries, mealtimes are still considered a social event rather than feasting. Mealtimes should be a happy, harmonious, comfortable, and relaxed occasion, but we tend to think of them today with respect to choice, volume, calories, and nutrition.

It is, however, possible to start viewing meals as an emotional experience in addition to a culinary one, and viewing the serving size on your plate as being proportionate to obtaining a feeling of emotional satisfaction. Stop worrying about food and stop worrying about the calories. Stop thinking about the numbers on the scale and stop treating food as if it were an enemy rather than something your body needs to maintain itself and its health at optimum levels.

The way to enjoy food is to start when you are shopping for it. Take more time and look at colors, textures, local food options, and varieties. You will soon discover that you do not have to think about a "balanced diet" if you view food in this way, because the diet will balance itself.

Although it may initially appear separate, your digestive system is strongly linked to your emotions. Eating is governed by the parasympathetic nervous system, and rest and digestion are intertwined. Becoming stressed about food, whether it is worrying about shopping for it, preparing it, cooking it, or the calories it contains, can actually trigger negative digestive effects.

As you chop foods up and prepare them, take time to think about the amount of spices and salt to add, and negotiate between healthy options and taste. Get the balance right and this will satisfy both your brain and emotions, as well as your stomach later. Allow your cooking process to make you and your family feel healthy, and make eating the meal something that brings everyone together.

Taking this approach affects your digestive system, which is dominated by the rest and digestion parasympathetic phase. If you go to a famous chef's restaurant, your brain and emotions are already harmonized, so when you see the nicely presented dish and taste the exquisite food, you feel really happy and relaxed right away—even without wine.

However, if you are endlessly concerned about the calories in every meal or worry about gaining weight, or start to discriminate good food from that which is bad, these concerns break down your meal-harmonizing process. Alternatively, if you eat a meal in an uncomfortable environment, you will feel indigestion building almost immediately. Notice, too, that if you eat at a restaurant that is not clean, then you will probably feel uncomfortable abdominal symptoms later, even if the food was actually great.

In reality, things can't always be perfect and your conditions for eating can be disrupted by factors such as a busy schedule and not having time to eat, or by suffering emotional hurt, when you will not have much of an appetite. Always try to regulate your daily eating habits because this is going to keep your hormonal system balanced.

RESETTING YOUR DIGESTIVE SYSTEM

Most of us realize that emotional stress usually affects our eating habits and digestive system. Whether you are a comfort eater in times of stress or simply have no appetite, there is a way to reset your digestive functions. Most people interpret comfort foods as being those they eat in times of stress. However, real comfort foods are the ones we enjoyed in childhood. Revert to childhood and avoid eating very hot or very cold meals. Avoid any excessively dark green vegetables, raw mushrooms, exotic foods, or alcohol. In fact, avoid anything you would not give to your one-year-old baby. Look instead to single-grained cereals, pureed sweet potato, or banana. Try to think of nurturing not your emotions, but your digestive system.

Whenever I was sick as a child, my grandmother made me rice porridge with ground beef and salt. After eating it, I always fell asleep for a few hours and then—magically—I was well enough to go back to school. Even now, whenever I do not feel well, I head straight to a Chinese or Korean restaurant to get congee (porridge) before setting off for home and a quiet lie-down.

Although we have discussed the parasympathetic and sympathetic nervous systems, what we have not mentioned yet is the enteric nervous system. The enteric nervous system runs from the esophagus to the anus and has more than five times the neurons than that of the spinal cord. It can also run independently of both the spinal cord and the brain; hence, you will find that the enteric nervous system is sometimes referred to as the second brain. The digestive system is activated by parasympathetic nerves that typically stimulate senses—such as seeing and smelling—resulting in the secretion of digestive hormones in the stomach. Emotions such as anger, fear, and anxiety may slow digestion because they stimulate the sympathetic nerves that supply the gastrointestinal tract, reducing any feelings of hunger.

The enteric nervous system controls motility (the contraction of the muscles that mix and propel contents in the gastrointestinal tract) through the small and large intestines, regulation of fluid exchange and local blood flow, regulation of gastric and pancreatic secretion, regulation of gastrointestinal endocrine cells, and defense reactions.

In my clinical experience, I find that patients with digestive issues have a corresponding issue with depression or anxiety, and most of these patients have experienced some kind of change in body shape. Additionally, for example, there is a significant relationship between abdominal surgery and strained back muscles in patients. Once the body's structural problem is identified and resolved, the symptoms are reduced.

AND YOU THOUGHT LOSING WEIGHT WAS SIMPLE?

I am well aware that all the information I have given you so far may seem daunting, but it is essential that you start to understand exactly what happens with respect to changing body shape, weight gain, and possible underlying health conditions. Remember that the body shape you desire should be the body shape that indicates that you, *as an individual*, are healthy. Weight loss and our diets are only small factors that can influence our body shape. Our health, both historical and current, the way we live our lives, and the way we think about living our lives all significantly affect not only our size and shape, but also our state of mind.

What I am going to share with you in the subsequent chapters are some alternative ideas for getting to where you *should* be, and understanding that looking like a catwalk model or a film star is not ideal for the great majority of people. We are who we are, but in all of us there is most likely a better way to treat our bodies, and that means getting them into the right shape for each of the different body types that I will discuss in detail later.

2

A First Look at the Meridian System in TCM

UNDERSTANDING THE ESSENTIALS (QI AND MERIDIAN)

Within traditional Chinese medicine (TCM), the meridian system is the path, sometimes called a channel network, through which the life energy known as Qi flows. We need to understand the meridian system and the body tissue functions and structures before we move on.

From a scientific perspective, this meridian system of energy paths has no direct correlation to modern medicine, since it cannot be seen, weighed, or measured from a scientific point of view, at least in accordance with current scientific research methods, and it is hard to prove in short papers.

Qi is all the key actions of a living organism: metabolism, homeostasis, breathing, heartbeat, blood circulation, inflammation, digestion, absorption, excretion, and so on. It also covers all biomechanical movements, including cell osmotic pressure, white blood cell migration from blood vessels to cells, skin pore closure action, sweating, intestinal peristalsis, hormonal negative feedback loop, human vitality, and muscle movement. Scientific research into the Qi mechanism encompasses biology, biochemistry, and biophysics.

Qi can be a "something" to someone who uses the word, depending on his or her understanding, but from my medical perspective, Qi is all kinds of bioactivity, but especially homeostasis, the ability to maintain a stable condition, the metabolic energy for the survival of a living organism, and the action of all organs, tissues, and skeletal muscle movement for the body's mechanical activities. All these systemic functions and by-products are explained by the one word *Qi*.

The meridian system has been known for centuries, and the body meridians show the current body conditions when observed carefully. We can reach and influence the internal organ systems through the meridian system in order to treat and prevent disorders. I use a number of manual treatment methods, such as acupuncture needles, moxibustion, cupping, gua sha, and hyperthermal methods. Of these, the acupuncture meridian is the

13

most important guideline for diagnosis and prognosis and for comparing before and after treatment.

Twelve main meridians are used in most acupuncture clinics for relieving ailments. There are also 8 extraordinary meridians, 12 divergent meridians, 12 muscle regions or meridians, and 12 cutaneous regions or meridians. The muscle and skin meridians can also be called a region because they indicate the connecting region rather than lines.

For body reshaping treatment, a muscle tendon regional meridian, a skin cutaneous regional meridian, and eight extraordinary meridians are used in my clinic. These meridians are explained in detail in Chapters 5 and 7.

OBESITY IS DEVELOPED STEP BY STEP

When we speak of fat, we tend to view it simply as a layer under the skin of our bodies, as something that is somehow distinct from other internal structures. Nothing could be further from the truth. Skin, fat, vessels, serous fluids, membranes, muscles, and organs all work together in harmony, so fat cannot be viewed as an isolated issue; it must be examined in the context of what is happening around it.

TCM defines a healthy condition as the balance between yin and yang, between a smooth Qi and blood circulation. When these conditions are disturbed, pathological symptoms occur, and being overweight or obese is considered the pathologic term *dampness*, which is mostly related to the spleen. This is further differentiated into two conditions: damp heat and damp cold.

Being overweight or obese and dampness in the body follow these steps:

1. Slow digestive system involving autonomic nervous system
2. Imbalance of internal cavity pressure with gas and body fluids
3. Edema due to muscle weakness and body fluid imbalance
4. Hormonal imbalance due to long-term congestion and imbalance of homeostasis

External trauma such as surgery and scarring can also affect Qi and blood circulation, which, in turn, can lead to the development of dampness.

SPLEEN FUNCTIONS IN TCM

The functions of the spleen are

- Transportation and transformation
- Controlling blood
- Dominating the muscles and four limbs
- The complex of the opening into the mouth and lips

Autonomic Nervous System and Spleen Function

When I began to consider the Chinese theories regarding the spleen in the context of their correlation to Western medicine, the question "What transport mechanism is used?" arose. The answer, it seemed, was simple. Serous (clear and watery) fluid came to mind. Serous fluid is glandular fluid found in most parts of the body cavities and is enriched with proteins, water, and sometimes enzymes. These fluids assist several body functions, such as digestion, respiration, and excretion.

When it comes to serous fluid, saliva is possibly the easiest example to use. The secretion of saliva can be stimulated by both the parasympathetic and sympathetic nervous systems. It is released by the salivary gland and contains an enzyme called amylase that helps digest carbohydrates. Under normal circumstances, watery saliva is stimulated by the parasympathetic nerve to facilitate digestion, but in situations of acute stress, saliva is stimulated by the sympathetic nervous system, which facilitates the respiration to inhibit the secretion of saliva.

When the body needs to detect stressors or outside dangers, it focuses the outside senses, such as listening and seeing, for a quicker response, and so the internal body senses, such as taste, become less active. When you are in a stressful situation, your breathing becomes shallow and you feel that things become quiet; this is a result of the sympathetic action of the bronchial passage dilating to increase respiration. Most people, although unsure why, immediately recognize the difference because when saliva is produced under stressful circumstances, it becomes thick and dry.

Transportation and Transformation of Spleen Function in TCM

The spleen connects to the stomach, both internally and externally. Food enters the stomach and is partially degraded by acid before being moved on toward the small intestine.

When the food has been degraded further and is considered pure, the spleen begins the process of transferring and transforming it into the nutritional Qi. The direction of the nutritional Qi flow is upward and it is sent to the heart and lungs. This is opposed to stomach Qi, which flows downward.

When the Qi passes the heart, it combines with prenatal Qi. In the lungs, it then blends with the air Qi and original Qi to form true Qi, which is then spread throughout the body. If this function is unimpaired, the Qi is strong, resulting in good digestion, smooth body movement, and moist extremities. When true Qi is impaired and weak, pathological symptoms arise. These manifest themselves in a variety of symptoms, including poor appetite, indigestion, loose stools, phlegm, and damp accumulation in the middle Jiao, which is located in the abdominal cavity area.

Dampness in Spleen Function Imbalance in TCM

In Chinese medicine, dampness refers to an accumulation of unhealthy fluids, most of which are obvious, for example, phlegm, pus, mucus, and other discharges. Fluids that we pass normally when we are healthy are not considered dampness, but some, particularly when they are located around the abdominal region, may not immediately strike us as dampness, but in fact are. For example, a localized swollen feeling in the lower back or side area from prolonged sitting—local congestions—can be considered dampness.

Extremities and Muscle: Spleen Function in TCM

The spleen is seen to dominate not only the muscles, but also the four limbs. If the spleen is weak, the muscles are not nourished and they become tired and weak. Often, contracted muscles are considered healthy and strong, but in fact, relaxed and soft muscles are regarded as healthy.

When you work out to build intense power, the muscle can be contracted and stretched at the same time. Moreover, fine detailed movements should be performed with distal muscles. Sufficient blood flow and body fluids are needed for healthy muscle condition. When you are relaxed, your salivary glands secrete more watery saliva that flows more easily toward your gut system and so affects your respiratory system by ensuring an unrestricted bronchial passage. You are able to breathe deeply in a diaphragmatic motion within the abdominal and thoracic cavity.

With regard to digestive function, I cannot overemphasize the importance of the flow of nutrients. Once absorbed, digestive nutrients in the blood and lymphatic vessels are transported toward the thoracic cavity to join the circulatory system. This functional movement is aided by the lower extremities' venous return pumps and diaphragmatic respiratory action. This means that your digestive system has not completed its task until the nutrients have been sent to the circulatory system. For this process, your body needs its musculoskeletal pump action and respiratory system function. So, light walking or strolling after a meal is recommended by TCM practitioners.

To reach a good nutritional state in the body, you need a balanced diet and a healthy digestive system, parasympathetic mode, musculoskeletal movements, diaphragmatic breathing, and heart action.

Diaphragm and Congestion in Abdominal Cavity

I then began to consider the spleen's upward movement as possibly corresponding with diaphragm drainage. The diaphragm has a system of lymphatic vessels that remove fluids and cells from the diaphragm itself, and it also plays a major role in the removal of fluid and cells from the pleura (the area where the lungs are situated) and peritoneal cavity, the fluid-filled gap between the walls of the abdomen and the organs in the abdomen.

When the diaphragm contracts correctly, several issues related to weight gain can be resolved. For example, congestion in the abdomen, effective transference of enzymes, and the transport of nutrients through the lymphatic vessels are not impeded.

We tend to separate organ functions into different specialties, such as gastrointestinal, gynecological, internist, cardiovascular, respiratory, neuroscience, and ear, nose, and throat (ENT). No doubt, such divisions allow for isolated in-depth knowledge within the specialties themselves; however, the functional flow connecting each body system has to be understood, allowing for optimal disorder prevention and health maintenance.

This provides us with the ideal contrast between Eastern and Western medicine, as the West concentrates on specialization, while the East focuses on the whole, or holistic, interpretation.

So, before we even consider the nature of the food we eat—if we are considering changing our body shape—we first have to ensure that our systems, with respect to gastrointestinal, diaphragm, autonomic nervous system, venous system, respiratory system, and respiratory muscles, are functioning optimally, because they work together, and if one aspect fails, disorder will result.

BODY CAVITIES AND BODY FLUIDS

The body has three major cavities containing visceral organs, and all are located in the torso. They comprise the thoracic cavity, abdominal cavity, and pelvic cavity. The organs within these cavities are protected by an intricate network of membranes and serous fluids. The different membranes also contain variable amounts of fat, and these, too, are attached to various muscles, most importantly the transverse abdominis and intercostal muscles. By altering tensions of connective tissue, both muscles play a key role in the body reshaping treatment and ridding the body of dampness.

Dampness, Edema, and Disorders

The body fluids are balanced by four different mechanisms, and if these all function correctly, body fluid will not accumulate because production and reabsorption take place at a constant rate. However, if even one of these mechanisms does not function normally, fluid can accumulate. In some cases, where plasma starts to accumulate outside of cells, the result is edema.

Although it might not initially seem important, the subject of edema is particularly relevant to body shape and our health in general, but not all edema is the same. One type—transudate edema—is caused by fluid moving out of the vessels and into the body cavity, and this is not linked to inflammatory conditions.

On the other hand, exudate edema is caused by a mass of cells and fluid that have seeped out of blood vessels or an organ and is related to inflammatory conditions. Transudate edema is most commonly linked to illnesses such as congestive heart failure and cirrhosis, but can also be associated with certain conditions, including chronic localized infections such as sinusitis, gastrointestinal malabsorption issues, and hypothyroidism. If this chronic transudate edema continues without intervention, people may misinterpret their weight gain as being due to unhealthy eating habits or a sedentary lifestyle.

San Jiao (Triple Burner) in TCM and Body Cavities

In TCM, there are corresponding organ systems with body cavities and serous fluid functions.

Each organ is not a single self-contained entity, but rather a functional energy system involved in regulating the activities of other organs responsible for the movement and transformation of various solids and fluids throughout the system. Composed of three parts, known as burners, each organ is associated with one of the body's three main cavities: thorax, abdomen, and pelvis. Ancient Chinese medical texts state, The upper burner controls intake, the middle burner controls transformation, the lower burner controls elimination.

The triple burner is also referred to as the San Jiao system in TCM and relates to the passage of heat and fluid through the body and the identification of disease according to the three burners.

This is often combined with TCM's four stages theory when diagnosing and treating an externally contracted disease caused by a wind–heat pathogen. Although the term *wind–heat* may seem unrelated to illness to Western minds, the analogy is quite simple: wind, cold, and heat can all bring bad, or pathogenic, organisms from outside into the body.

Upper Jiao includes the heart, lungs, and pericardium organs, and its pathogenic patterns are usually wind–heat as a sign of upper Jiao organ inflammation and infection with dry-heat factors.

The middle Jiao includes the spleen, stomach, gall bladder, and liver organs, and the pattern of the pathogen presents with severe damp and heat signs. The lower Jiao includes the small and large intestines, the kidneys, and the bladder, and the pathogenic pattern is more observable in the chronic stages of dry-heat inflammation.

These are very important concepts for treating a number of different body types in body reshaping, because the pathogenic patterns among upper, lower, and middle burners exhibit different inflammatory conditions for dry-heat and damp-heat patterns.

Unlike a sluggish digestive system caused by an autonomic nervous system and exhibiting a cold pathogenic pattern, the congestion of fluids in the abdominal cavity can result from the external heat pathogens and dampness.

This clue brings about a different view on abdominal obesity, which can be classified as a chronic allergic reaction due to sensitivity to external pathogens, and sluggish digestive system obesity induced by chronic stress. These patterns are the cornerstones for type P and type T.

HEALTHY HABITS AND CIRCADIAN RHYTHM

Many of us "follow nature," and our body clock and habits are created by the repetition (with mental association) of behaviors performed automatically following frequent past actions; lack of thought is the key factor in differentiating between habitual and nonhabitual actions. Healthy eating habits and regular physical activity are important to well-being, and even small changes in the right direction can improve your health. Improper eating, sleeping, or even bad breathing habits can lead to health problems.

Research has established that we start to form habits around the ages of five to seven years old. It is therefore essential that by the time children reach this age, parents and those in authority have been active role models to their children with healthy eating, sleeping, and physical activity, because these habits can last a lifetime. As discussed earlier, mirroring the habits of children can positively affect adults in their own lives. This is not just about what we eat, but also about improving our health by mirroring their posture, behavior, and lifestyle.

With regard to learned behavior, four healthy habits are essential:

- Good nutrition and a nontoxic diet
- Quality sleep
- Movement and exercise
- Self-regulated stress management

Outside of our socially learned habits relating to social, cultural, and environmental influences, we are also governed by our body clock. This ticks in accordance with nature and affects certain behaviors and functions relating to day and night, the seasons, a grumbling stomach requiring food, growing, and of course, aging.

Ultimately, and more particularly when it comes to the natural law of time, we find that our lives and health are made much easier if we accept and work with the natural laws, rather than fight against them. The natural law of time means that our body responds to biological time, a measurement on the 24-hour timescale, and is regulated by a circadian timing mechanism.

CIRCADIAN RHYTHMS AND THE MERIDIAN CLOCK

Circadian rhythms are controlled by the body's biological clock, which has a rhythmic pattern coinciding with the Earth's 24-hour cycle around the sun. However, there are not only 24-hour cycles; for example, a menstrual cycle is about 28–30 days, pregnancy is about 9 months, a gastric phase is between 3 and 4 hours. These circadian rhythms affect nearly every body function and activity we perform, and according to Chinese medicine, our body parts function optimally at certain preset times.

Viewing this from a TCM perspective, the meridian clock cycle is also known as the horary cycle, as Qi flows through the meridians, one by one (Figure 2.1). There are 12 meridians, and the duration of the Qi is two hours in each one, so each meridian experiences two cycles each day. When the Qi flow in a certain meridian seeks to increase the Qi within the corresponding organ system, energy can be increased.

- 1:00–3:00 a.m.—liver (foot—Jueyin)
- 3:00–5:00 a.m.—lung (hand—Taiyin)
- 5:00–7:00 a.m.—large intestine (hand—Yangming)
- 7:00–9:00 a.m.—stomach (foot—Yangming)
- 9:00–11:00 a.m.—spleen (foot—Taiyin)
- 11:00 a.m.–1:00 p.m.—heart (hand—Shaoyin)
- 1:00–3:00 p.m.—small intestine (hand—Taiyang)
- 3:00–5:00 p.m.—urinary bladder (foot—Taiyang)
- 5:00–7:00 p.m.—kidney (foot—Shaoyin)
- 7:00–9:00 p.m.—pericardium (hand—Jueyin)

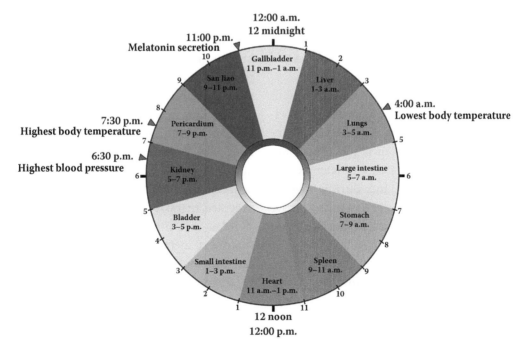

FIGURE 2.1
Horary clock.

- 9:00–11:00 p.m.—triple burner (San Jiao) (hand—Shaoyang)
- 11:00 p.m.–1:00 a.m.—gall bladder (foot—Shaoyang)

SLEEP AND WAKEFULNESS: HOMEOSTATIC BALANCE

If we take a closer look at the day and night cycles, it is clear that sunlight is the master key for biological clock rhythms. Another strongly influencing factor is the hormone melatonin, which is released in response to darkness and influences phases of the circadian rhythm.

During the day, most organs are involved in catabolic reactions such as producing body heat, moving muscles, and other essential functions. At night, anabolic reactions are dominant, and they are involved in healing wounds, restoring energy, and the growth of children. The balance between anabolism and catabolism is also regulated by circadian rhythms, and that is why we feel swollen and bloated after a sleepless night.

During sleep, most systems in humans and animals are in an anabolic state, building up the immune, nervous, and skeletomuscular systems. Sleep is very important as anabolism needs energy to later excrete the waste products, and during a good sleep, the skeletal muscles and sphincter are relaxed, preparing us for a productive bowel movement in the morning.

Many things can disrupt the meridian clock cycle: working night shift, jet lag, and delayed or advanced sleep patterns. These may result in insomnia, excessive daytime sleepiness, or even both. Eating too much, not eating enough, and eating late at night also disturb sleep patterns. These circadian rhythm disorders are associated with an increased risk of accidents, and they impair quality of life by inducing problems such as weight gain or local body congestion.

PARALLELS BETWEEN ASIAN AND WESTERN MEDICINE

Although it may initially appear not to be the case, there are many parallels between Asian and Western medical practices. In the West, *kinesiology* is the term used for the scientific study of human movement. This is a very broad field and incorporates many elements, from rehabilitation methods to biomechanics. In Asia, acupuncture and moxibustion treatments are well known and widely used in the same contexts, for example, neuromuscular disabilities, including conditions that affect the spinal cord, peripheral nerves, neuromuscular junctions, and muscles. Acupuncture integrates Eastern and Western medicine and may use electro-acupuncture or laser acupuncture as alternatives to the widely accepted manual "needling." Furthermore, TCM is not limited to one modality or treatment method, but may also incorporate moxibustion, cupping, Chinese tui na massage, or gua sha.

3

Who Can Benefit from This Treatment?

WEIGHT LOSS OR DIET LIFE VERSUS MY LIFE

As most people will testify, when any health issue arises, so does the subject of diet and exercise. Our lifestyle and habits usually come under the microscope as a first port of call. Diet, exercise, or a general change of habits will often be recommended to someone who suffers health issues, wants to improve his or her body shape, or simply wants to lose weight. Yet, many people who embark upon a regimen rarely experience long-term success, even if it is successful in the short term.

One problem revolves around the fact that rather than making small, staggered changes, we are usually thrust, or thrust ourselves, into a frantic pattern of sudden rearrangements relating to eating, physical activities, sleeping habits, and attitude. The goal becomes getting "healthy" or "fit" without us having any real understanding of what this actually means. All this change and activity are usually driven by one single factor: our goal. The goal is the finish line, a factor based on time or quantity and one that is decided upon before we even embark on our new healthy living regimen.

Initially, once the decision is made to lose weight or improve health, there is a feeling of satisfaction and challenge. We start to mark off weight loss on a calendar or record how many calories we are eating. We note how much protein or carbohydrates we need and the types of foods that are better for us. And, during this period of commitment, the feeling of satisfaction increases—we are on our way to achieving our *goal*.

Unfortunately, the goal always has a finish line—whether it is successful or not. Usually, we determine our success by how much weight we have lost, how much our muscles have developed, how good our body looks, how far blood sugar levels have fallen, or even how successful we have been in cutting down favorite foods or alcohol. These are all possible ways of feeling achievement and reaching our goal. But, what many people fail to realize is that the real goal is not to achieve their aim, but to go past it—to finish what you embarked upon and experience relief and satisfaction in knowing you are on your way to a conclusion and getting on with life.

What happens then? For many of us, several months after the achievement of our goal—no matter how successful we have been—similar health issues may arise or our body shape changes again, and for no good reason. Even though many maintain a commitment to exercise or establishing more healthy eating habits, the body shape we acquired or the health benefits we expected simply do not remain.

If you are one of these people, this chapter will go a long way to helping you understand how you need to correct your body condition before you can improve or maintain your health. This is especially relevant to those who have suffered physical trauma, illness, or a similar situation, and where simple diet and exercise are failing to produce the required benefits.

BODY RESHAPING AND SUCCESSFUL HEALTH REGIMENS

Body reshaping can benefit many people, but more particularly those who have issues with poor posture due to muscle dystrophy (muscle atrophy resulting from illness as opposed to muscular dystrophy, an illness in its own right), tissue adhesion, or chronic pain, particularly with numbness.

Correcting the posture is a common concern among patients and health practitioners. The relationship between poor posture and internal or external health issues has been acknowledged for a long time. Sometimes doctors use exercise, manipulation, or surgery to help correct a postural problem that it is not too severe. Although I use the term *posture*, and this may seem distinct from any health issues, we only have to look at how athletes often employ

the services of physiotherapists to correct potential or actual problems. This is a clear example of a postural problem causing physical issues, which is recognized by most people.

In Chapter 1, I suggested you examine your posture and try to assess if it was correct and, if not, what you think is wrong with it. This is not about whether you find your body shape or figure attractive, but simply about how you position yourself when performing a variety of activities and actions. Does your posture reflect a picture of health or otherwise?

I also mentioned in Chapter 1 that good posture could be identified as the body taking the stance that consumes the least energy against gravity, whether we are standing, sitting, or moving. No matter what we do, like the athletes who are highly aware of posture, we should realize that an optimal posture exists for every movement we make, whether we are going about our daily activities or performing repetitive actions.

When we have our body posture assessed, it is usually from a static standing position. When standing, the body form is determined by our spine and attention is paid to thoracic curvature, lumbar curvature, and sacral or sacrum hip angles. But this type of assessment has its limitations because the "motion makers" are the hands and legs rather than the spine and trunk. You may have observed that when you walk, you swing your arms—they do not remain static. In fact, arm movement when walking is so significant that immobile arms can be an important indicator of several serious conditions that involve spinal cord issues. So the spinal posture is influenced by how we move our arms and legs, and these can change, depending on whether our posture is correct, or it may change depending on the injury we have sustained. For example, you may have sprained an ankle, yet when you stand still, your posture is still correct; but what happens when you try to move? Hip and back muscles are affected by walking and moving on this painful ankle because it affects the spine and the spinal muscle to the brain. So the way we use our extremities should always be considered when evaluating the correct posture in movement.

Diagnosis from the six body types and muscle and skin meridian treatments is designed to balance body postural performance. This is because when it comes to correcting posture, we do not focus only on the spine or muscles, but on the entire body formation that contributes to movement and on the connection between the functions and systems, both externally and internally.

If we view the body shape as a constructed building, the bones and muscles are the foundation of the structural body shape. Nevertheless, we still need to consider the total involvement of the organism, no matter how small or seemingly insignificant. Because living organisms are constantly moving either internally or externally, they are transformed by actions such as breathing, intestinal motility, skin cell regeneration, cell migration, and myriad other autonomic functions, even when physically immobile.

Even orthodox medicine cannot always accurately assess the root cause of a problem, despite a wealth of available technical equipment. For example, if you have a splinter in the sole of your foot, you cannot run. Or maybe a small paper cut on your finger temporarily disables the hand. But an x-ray will reveal nothing too severe. The bone will still be intact and the finger structure will be normal, despite the fact that the splinter or cut, quite possibly, can affect your movements and ultimately your posture.

With regard to posture and repetitive daily actions, each movement should take into consideration your job, work environment, and habits. Normally, when we move, the most active movements are primarily those that affect the extremities, and they are the ones on which most repeat actions are made. This repeated action makes maximum use of one muscle group and minimum use of another, which results in the least-used muscle group becoming weakened and lengthened, and which can detrimentally affect posture. The problem is compounded further because, in addition to the lymphatic flow being affected in this region, the venous returns also depend on muscle flexibility when contracting.

Clinical observations prove that localized puffy and swollen areas of congestion can be found on the surface of a lengthened muscle, even when inflammation is not present. This makes it difficult to palpate muscles by hand because the area concerned usually feels tight and hard enough to actually obscure the muscle itself. This problem is particularly prevalent in areas such as the triceps on the arm, the latissimus dorsi muscle on the upper back, and the breast area.

SUBCUTANEOUS FAT

What we can learn from all this is that problems arising from poor posture are not simply related to muscle and bone misalignment, but involve many other autonomic functions of the body. Yet, even outside of these issues, we also have to consider the skin itself and, of course, subcutaneous fatty tissues.

Problems involving subcutaneous fat usually affect the inner thigh, armpit, and lower back where adipose tissue is found, which then become congested and affect the range of motion. These areas can also present with skin discoloration and stretch marks on the tendon and fascia of contracted muscles. This may result in flabby deposits and hard mass types, but most patients find that whatever the type, it affects voluntary and involuntary movement.

My six body types muscle meridian treatment takes the approach of looking at the outer skin, subcutaneous tissues, and myofascial problems in that order. This means that before aligning the skeletal muscles, the skin and any local fatty tissue congestion need to be loosened. Once the outer skin and fatty tissues are loosened, the lengthened muscles are treated with a muscle meridian needling technique prior to treating the contracted muscle group. Because the muscle meridian focus is on the soft to hard and small to large muscle groups, close observation of movement is very important and patients may be asked to perform soft and slow motions to enable accurate assessment.

Today, a primary focus of our lives is on excellence. We have grown accustomed to going further, doing things more quickly, achieving greater results, and exceeding or performing to the extreme. Unfortunately, the attitude we have toward our body is no different. Instead of excess, we need to look at moderation and neutrality to find our own individual points of balance.

of great joy for all family members, for the mother it can result in a variety of problems. After childbirth, the speed at which a mother's body recovers can vary dramatically because each woman has different genetics, health issues, personal situations, and tolerance for her condition. If you ask most mothers to compare their bodies before pregnancy with how they are after it, most will agree that their body has not fully recovered.

Again, we must realize that childbirth is not the finish line. The heavy, loaded body does not simply change because a mother is no longer pregnant. Taking care of a new and growing baby, when your body is already exhausted from the birth and nine months of body change, is a difficult job.

New mothers should receive postpartum care until their body can maintain the correct posture and function. In several countries, this is standard practice and is an accepted fact. As the baby begins to grow, the mother may find she has sudden weight gain, back pain, and symptoms of chronic fatigue. This problem usually increases when the baby begins to gain weight and is able to move around on his or her own, and it may become even more pronounced when the baby reaches the toddler stage. Frequent bending of the back and carrying a heavy, playful baby can be an overload on the mother's arms and shoulders. This is why most women who have delivered a child or children find that their body shape changes, not only during pregnancy, but also in the years that follow.

POSTCHILDBIRTH COMPLICATIONS

Although pregnancy and childbirth are natural phenomena and usually a source

CAESAREAN SECTION

Delivery by caesarean or C-section, like most surgical procedures, involves an incision of the skin. Although most surgical wounds appear to be completely closed after a procedure and heal over several days or months, this is not always true. Regardless of the surgery performed, complications arising from it do not surface immediately or even after several months, which makes it difficult to directly trace any complications from operations. The human body has multiple layers of tissue, and during a C-section, the following layers are cut in order to perform the procedure: subcutaneous fat, rectus sheath, rectus abdominis, abdominal peritoneum, pelvic peritoneum, and uterine muscle. Currently, most C-section procedures involve a 15-centimeter transverse line incision near the pubis.

Yet most patients have little idea of what their surgical procedure involves and the operation itself seems simple enough—after all, most women undergoing a C-section usually spend only two or three days longer in the hospital than women who have delivered normally. This is despite it being unlike many other surgical procedures, and in many ways more complicated because it involves the visceral and gastrointestinal peritoneum and the inguinal area.

In my clinical observation, though the scar of a C-section may appear clear and have no obvious complications, I often find that the area under the skin has a palpable mass. Additionally, the area around the lower abdomen can be bloated and larger than that which surrounds it. This affects many women, and they mention that they want to lose fat from both the lower abdomen and hip regions.

ADHESION-RELATED DISORDER

Adhesion-related disorders (ARDs) refer to the condition of internal abdominal organs that are attached abnormally. They may develop following most types of surgical procedures. Moreover, many of the problems related to such adhesions are asymptomatic and difficult to diagnose, or they may be simply overlooked because the symptoms are so variable. This can result in other organ complications, such as idiopathic infertility, bowel obstruction, chronic abdominal pain, pelvic pain, leg pain, and many other conditions.

If an adhesion-related disorder is severe, it can involve endometriosis, interstitial cystitis, painful intercourse, and irritable bowel syndrome and result in an inability to work or maintain family or social relationships. Abdominal pains from such adhesions are a common complaint, but most surgeons do not perform remedial surgery unless the patient suffers from a bowel obstruction or severe secondary inflammation.

Patients do not attend my clinic on the recommendation of a clinician to have a diagnosed adhesion disorder treated, but I have treated patients to assist in correcting pelvic and abdominal cavity and hip and waist alignment and, in doing so, have discovered abdominal scars. The scars vary but usually indicate any of the following procedures: appendectomy, ovariectomy, liver cell biopsy, laparoscopy, C-section, hysterectomy, and many other surgical procedures.

Surgery to the lower abdomen appears to affect the small intestine, urinary bladder, and uterus. Common clinical observations include the shape of the body while standing. The overall standing posture is quite distinctive and is somewhat similar to a sitting position, with the pelvis tilted anteriorly. This type of posture can also be seen on people who spend substantial periods sitting at a desk.

These conditions are classified as the M2 body type and whole-body observations are required. A chronic adhesion-related discomfort on the abdomen may influence an entirely different location, such as the face, neck, foot, or even eye muscles. Sometimes an adhesion on the lower abdomen may restrict movement in the lower extremities, and at other times, one side may be more affected than the other. For example, one leg may be markedly affected when the body is in motion, which deforms the upper body posture because it is compensating for the problem.

FUNCTIONAL GASTROINTESTINAL DISORDERS

Functional gastrointestinal disorders (FGIDs) are disorders of the digestive system characterized by pain or discomfort, such as irritable bowel syndrome, functional dyspepsia, and other conditions associated with many reports of abdominal discomfort, but in which pain is not the dominant symptom. Psychological factors such as depression, anxiety, panic, and posttraumatic stress disorder are all associated with these symptoms.

Eating too rapidly, discomfort eating, and particularly eating when angry have long been considered bad habits for the digestive system. Delayed bowel movements or bowel movements encouraged by laxatives also have a negative influence. After eating, mild walking and taking time to relax are known to help digestion and are highly recommended.

Many people suffer digestive discomfort and irregular bowel movements, but unless the pain is severe or there is acute vomiting with blood present, little is usually done and the milder symptoms are ignored. In most cases, sufferers will self-medicate and take over-the-counter medication rather than trouble their clinician with symptoms that are indicative of discomfort rather than illness.

When most functional gastrointestinal disorders are investigated, no demonstrable cause is found. Symptoms may be similar to those of angina, but cardiac investigations are normal. A patient may have extreme heartburn but does not respond to acid suppressants. They may also undergo an esophageal pH study, the results of which are often negative. Epigastric pain often results in normal endoscopy findings and gastrointestinal symptoms with no organic cause.

Some patients that presented with FGID had existing chronic pain prior to their diagnosis and quite often simply lived with it by using some form of suppressants to make it tolerable. One of my patients had functional dyspepsia for five years. She had a blood test, ultrasound scan, endoscopy, and colonoscopy, all of which revealed nothing and resulted in an functional disorder (FD) diagnosis.

She visited my clinic for gastrointestinal resuscitation (GIR) treatment, and on examination, I found her pelvic and hip areas were markedly swollen, particularly in the iliotibial (IT) band area. She felt that she had gained weight and wore larger size trousers, and she wanted to lose weight. I explained the body types and problems associated with them and she agreed to try to correct the problem.

The patient explained that she had fallen when skiing several years before and, since then, had experienced pain in the hip. However, she went on to say that the pain had recently disappeared. But, while palpating the hip muscle gently with my hand, she became distressed and expressed extreme pain. I noted that the pain was primarily confined to the gluteus medius and tensor fascia latae muscles. The skin in those areas also had stretch marks and tension. This patient is typical of those who have major pain symptoms in the abdominal region, but the true source of their pain remains hidden for a long time.

This, I believe, is why some patients appear sensitive to certain pain while they are actually suffering from chronic discomfort due to the true injury. Chronic distress or pain sensation from the lower extremities can result in digestive issues. In these cases, patients usually have low tolerance of pain and a releasing method such as GIR is performed. In this particular case, the patient had better digestion after several sessions of acupuncture than prior to her injury.

MAJOR SCARS

These include recent scars, surgery, walking-gait deformity from pain, and so on. The body has an amazing ability to adapt relative to performing any difficult task if given time and repeated often enough. Rehabilitation, which includes healing from minor scars and recovery from ailments, injury, or major surgery, comes under adaptive abilities. However, the process of healing can create other physical issues that manifest after several months, or even years, because the body has been putting all its efforts into healing and recovery after a trauma.

When the skin is damaged, scar tissue starts to form on the underlying epithelium, yet the overall process of wound healing begins with inflammation, angiogenesis, migration and proliferation of fibroblasts, and scar formation—connective tissue remodeling.

Types of Scar

There are many different types of scars, including contracture scars from burns. Keloid scars are raised above the skin and tend to be purple in color as they produce more collagen. Atrophic scars are depressed into the skin and are typical of the pitting of adolescent acne. Hypertrophic scars are raised slightly above the skin with discoloration, but not to the same extent as keloid scars.

The most common scars are stretch marks, also called striae, which appear on the body during pregnancy or sudden growth during adolescence. Stretch mark scars are not the result of injury, but are caused by the skin stretching rapidly. The locale of the stretch mark is very important in relating the internal situation to the six body types treatment.

Both hypertrophic and keloid scars are the result of an abnormal healing response with excessive collagen deposits accumulating relative to normal wounds. A hypertrophic scar is raised, red, and nodular but remains within the confines of the original skin damage. Keloids occur due to abnormalities of scar formation usually occurring at sites of injury or inflammation. They differ from hypertrophic scars in their extension beyond the original injury site.

Burn scarring is differentiated according to the degree of damage to the skin. First-degree burns involve only the epidermis. Second-degree damage involves the superficial or deep dermis, and third degree extends to the subdermal tissues. Initial burn scars are hypertrophic until they start to contract and pull the skin and tissue together. Tightness in such scars results in relative immobility, particularly in the morning. Contracture after a burn injury is common on the shoulders, elbows, and knees, the most commonly affected joints. Included are areas of the tendon and ligament, as well as aponeurotic areas, which are poorly vascularized.

Traditional Chinese medicine (TCM) treats burn scars by first removing the toxins that have been incorporated into the affected area. First, the scar is anesthetized using acupuncture. Then it is treated with moxibustion therapy, including the moxa cream gua sha. This reconnects subcutaneous blood vessels to cutaneous muscles and facilitates subcutaneous lymph function. Loosening the scar also helps to open the gap between the scar and the underlying tissue.

Stretch Marks

Stretch marks can be horizontal or vertical scars. Their color tone is different from that of the surrounding area, and they are usually formed during pregnancy, in growing adolescents, or with sudden weight or muscle gain. Rarely are these stretch marks or striae, as they are termed medically, considered worthy of treatment because the problem is purely aesthetic rather than injurious.

The severity of stretch marks differs and usually only becomes recognizable after delivery or sudden weight loss; they are similar to hypertrophic scars. However, if the local cutaneous lymphatic vessels are not functioning properly, then neither are the arterial pulsations or muscle contractions, and the area will appear swollen. In these cases, the internal congestion and muscle fibers should be treated first because

the underlying tissue is also stretched and scarred. This happens particularly in specific regions such as the armpit, lower back area, and inner thigh. Once these areas are restored to functionality, there is the added benefit of the body looking slimmer.

CELLULITE

Cellulite is a condition that occurs in women and men. It results in skin having a dimpled, lumpy appearance and is most noticeable on the buttocks and thighs. It usually appears after puberty. Many women try a variety of methods to reduce the appearance of cellulite, but because it is caused by a misalignment between the leg and pelvic area and involves the skin, subcutaneous tissue, muscle, facia, and bone, they are rarely successful. The reason cellulite is more common in women than in men is precisely because the male and female pelvic structures are different. In a female, the pelvis is broad and tilted forward, as it is adapted for childbearing, whereas in the male, it is less severely angled, deep, and narrower to support heavy lifting. For this reason, the bone in the pelvis is thicker in men than it is in women.

Because of the difference in the organ structure and pelvis shape in women, both necessary for childbearing, the underlying muscles and tissues differ too—making women more susceptible to cellulite.

PERIPHERAL NEUROPATHIES

The symptoms of peripheral neuropathy are pain, weakness, numbness, and deficit of motor skills caused by damage to the peripheral nerves, usually in the distal areas, such as in the hands and feet. Peripheral neuropathy arises as a result of inflammation, infections, trauma, alcohol, toxic substance accumulations, genetic causes, and metabolic problems such as diabetes mellitus.

Since the peripheral nervous system includes sensory, motor, and autonomic nerves, the symptoms can vary widely, depending on the nerve involved. If the sensory nerve is damaged, numbness and tingling will gradually develop. There may also be a stabbing or burning sensation or extreme sensitivity to touch. If the motor nerve is affected, coordination skills will be diminished and muscles may become weak or even paralyzed. Moreover, if autonomic nerves are damaged, heat intolerance may result, as well as problems with sweat glands, skin pores, bowel movement, urination, and digestion.

Painful peripheral neuropathies are usually accompanied by psychological disturbances that may include sleep disorders, mood swings, lack of energy, and difficulty in concentrating, to name a few.

It is common in clinical findings that many diseases affecting the peripheral nervous system produce negative neurological symptoms or signs. This is due to peripheral nervous system damage, and although it causes pain initially, eventually the damaged nerve fiber ceases to carry the information and the sense of pain.

In overweight and obese patients, this loss of sensitivity is usually easily identified, particularly in the lower extremities, where the stretched skin shows a distinct loss. These patients tend to feel more pain in ligaments and tendons, such as the plantar fasciitis, and knees, which have little or no stretched skin.

In TCM, these pathological symptoms are diagnosed as damp and phlegm blocking the Qi and blood circulation, and there are many clinical studies providing information on treating peripheral neuropathy with acupuncture. Yet, since acupuncture is only part of the many treatment methods and can vary in itself by issues as simple as the different needles that can be used, the evidence relating to clinical experimentation is rarely fully explained.

TCM suggests that if the problem is located in the peripheral skin regions, the cutaneous meridian using a subcutaneous needle, such as the plum blossom, should be selected. An alternative treatment uses moxibustion in that area to facilitate circulation. Cupping and gua sha can also be added to the treatment plan, using an herbal formula recommended for internal organ balance. Even though acupuncture is renowned as a pain treatment, the regimen varies according to each patient's needs. However, this is rarely applied in research, as standardized treatments are often used to enable replication of approach.

EMOTIONAL EXPRESSION BY THE BODY

Our gestures, actions, and facial expressions are merely physical representations of our emotions and thoughts. Often, physical posture or actions reveal what we are actually thinking despite our efforts to suppress them. For example, if you are angry but do not want to reveal it, you may hold your breath, clasp your hands tightly, or tense your shoulders or mouth. Let's face it, if you are angry with your boss, you don't dance round him like a butterfly.

Yet, often the physical action is a response initiated by the nervous system. For example, people clasp their hands because it brings the blood into the hand to ready the muscles there. It is symbolic of fight or flight or, in this particular case, fight.

When someone detects danger, the sympathetic nervous system responds by focusing attention on the eyes and ears and the mouth closes. Your body is in a state of readiness and has to be fully alert (Figure 3.1). Imagine a boxer's posture—chin down, teeth clenched, arms in front to protect the face, eyes open wide, and the body bending forward—the typical Incredible Hulk.

Alternatively, consider a yoga posture for relaxing: the eyes are closed, the palms open, and the legs loose (Figure 3.2).

When we examine the posture of a person sitting at a computer, listening through earphones, or talking on the phone, it closely resembles the posture of the boxer. The whole scenario suggests tension, and when our body is tense, so is our digestive tract. Then illnesses such as digestive problems, temporomandibular joint (TMJ), anxiety, depression, or sleep disorders may occur.

TMJ

When your head is tilted upwards, it is easy to close your eyes and open your mouth. If your head is tilted down, it is easier to keep your eyes open and your mouth closed.

Like the brain, head muscles enable balance between the right and left side of the body. The temporomandibular joint is unique, and the two sides usually work together whenever we talk, laugh, eat, chew, or even breathe.

The TMJ is also one of the first joints a new baby uses when it sucks, smiles, or cries. The facial muscles and the TMJ are central to the way babies express their feelings.

But once we have learned to control our emotions and expressions as required in our respective social and cultural groups, we can disguise or suppress our emotions and do not display our genuine emotions to others. Yet, the TMJ can reveal our true thoughts and emotions.

Mastication is the chewing action that moves the TMJ and involves many other muscles and fasciae. Once we start to chew,

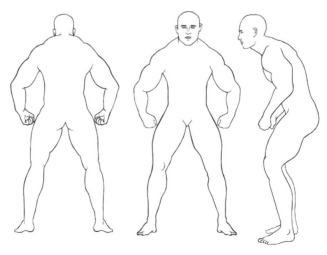

FIGURE 3.1
Muscle-tensed posture.

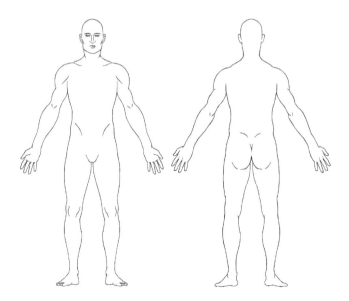

FIGURE 3.2
Standing posture.

saliva is secreted from salivary glands located on the sides of the face and lower jaw. The three pairs of major salivary glands are the parotid, which is the largest gland located in each cheek over the jaw in front of the ears; the submandibular, which is located at the back of the mouth on both sides of the jaw; and the sublingual glands, which are located under the floor of the mouth. Secreting saliva is an autonomic reflex that is also stimulated by the gustatory nerve.

As I observed TMJ problems in patients, I began to find that the problem, in many cases, is not from the joint of the temporomandibular itself, but from the parotid gland area, or simple tightness due to lymphatic fluids collecting in the same region.

Temporomandibular joint disorders (TMDs) are defined as a subgroup of craniofacial pain problems that involve the TMJ, masticatory muscles, and associated head and neck musculoskeletal structures. It is not just a local joint problem, and the pain or discomfort is often localized to the jaw, TMJ, and muscles of mastication.

If the symptoms are accompanied by joint sounds and corresponding locking, a feeling of dislocation, pain, and or any degenerative joint changes identified by x-ray, the disorder is related to specific problems in the temporomandibular joint. However, even though the problem is with the joints themselves, it will have a secondary effect on the surrounding muscles.

If the symptoms are primarily related to muscle pain and spasms, the problems are more likely to be of a myofascial origin. Since the face has many muscles and fascia that connect with one another from the neck and trunk, the pain may be triggered by the dysfunctional region and transmitted to the face. This condition is common in patients who are physically and mentally stressed, either temporarily or chronically.

This category of patient is usually classified as M1 and P in the body type groups.

In many cases of cervical spinal dysfunction relating to the spinal column, vertebrae, ligaments, or corresponding muscles, the majority of symptoms in the jaw will be referred pain arising from such problems. Again, this type of case is different from myofascial disorders and is classified as type M3.

BRUXISM

Many people suffer from bruxism but do not realize it. It is defined as the forced clenching or grinding of teeth during sleep or even when awake. It can often lead to dental problems and damage in a much larger proportion of the population than most people are aware. It is now known to occur in 15% of children and in a massive 75% of adults, yet the etiology is not fully understood, and several possible causes have been considered. Possible causes include the following: occlusal discrepancies, abnormal bony structures in the orofacial region, sleep arousal response, smoking, alcohol consumption, drug use, stress, personality type, and dopaminergic system disturbances.

I have had patients with concurrent symptoms of bruxism and oromandibular dystonia (forceful contractions of the face, jaw, or tongue), accompanied by severe tics. Whether coincidentally or not, most of these patients also have gastrointestinal problems relating to abdominal muscle tension arising from spinal muscle imbalance. I discovered that treating abdominal tension produced better results than acupuncture treatment in correcting this problem. Where craniofacial disorders also resulted in pain, a gentle approach of loosening the problem areas with a warm medium also met with considerable success.

DEPRESSION AND ANXIETY

Depression and anxiety are reflected physically, despite the fact that emotional conditions are subjective. When depressed, although we may feel sad, low, or weepy, we also have physical issues, such as disturbed sleep patterns, weight changes, lack of motivation, and decreased energy levels. In contrast, patients with manic symptoms of anxiety may have expansive or irritable moods, are easily angered, may be physically aggressive, suffer sleep disturbances, experience agitation, have racing thoughts, and experience increased levels of energy despite continually pushing themselves. Both depression and anxiety usually arise from psychosocial factors such as stress in combination with genetic and biochemical issues. The latter cause, of course, can be altered once the problems are treated successfully.

When I first trained in traditional Chinese medicine, the most fascinating part of the theory was the relationship among the organs, emotions, and disorders. Although the five basic emotions—joy, sadness, fear or fright, anger, and worry or pensiveness— are simply expressions of feelings, I learned that if the emotional state is extreme or of any duration, it may result in damage to the internal organs. Today, this concept is not limited to TCM; it is also accepted in orthodox medicine, as evidence has been offered that emotional disturbances can affect gut motility. Yet, in TCM, we have known for a long time that organs can be affected by lingering too long on one emotion. For example, too much thinking slows down the digestive system.

In TCM, certain organs and emotions are paired: lungs and sadness, heart and joy, liver and anger, spleen and worry or pensiveness, and kidneys and fear or fright. From a clinical perspective, it was difficult for me to attribute the pathologic influence of emotions on organ function because by the time I met patients, they already had systemic dysfunctions and I could not assume that the foundation was emotional. But, interestingly, patients who have specific organ dysfunctions tend to have emotional expressions that accompany them. For example, when there is tightness of the upper abdominal region and pulsation from a stress-induced situation, accompanying symptoms usually include indigestion, fatigue, muscle tightness, and anxiety. I found that once the tension was relieved, the symptoms were reduced, especially those of anxiety. It would seem that when the physical problems are resolved, the emotional issues are resolved simultaneously.

MEDICATION HISTORY COMPLICATIONS: ALLERGY MEDICATION

Often changes in the body are not acute, but creep up gradually. Body change is not always instantaneous, but gradually builds up due to delayed healing. The body classifications of P, T, and S, explained in Chapter 5, reflect how physical and mental stress can affect the autonomic nervous system and the hormonal system. The disturbances to the homeostasis of the body can often be expressed by allergic reactions, thyroid dysfunction, menstrual irregularity, sudden weight gain, and other, often diverse and deferred, reactions. Allopathic medicine often simply suppresses such symptoms. Yet, numerous medications may

result in weight gain for many of the patients to whom they are prescribed. For example, psychiatric and neurological treatments such as antidepressants, steroid hormones, antidiabetic drugs, antihistamines, and antihypertensive agents can result in weight gain. Also, other treatments obtained over the counter, such as some nutritional supplements and allergy treatments, can have the same effect. Obviously, if you wish to reshape your body, it is wise to be aware of the treatments that can result in weight gain and consequently impede weight loss.

OBESITY

The World Health Organization (WHO) has recognized obesity as a global epidemic disorder since 1997, and the prevalence of obesity in the United States was 35.7% in 2010. The U.S. National Health and Nutrition Examination Survey (NHANES) estimated that two out of every five adults in the United States will be obese by 2015.

Obesity and being overweight are not considered a disease in themselves until the effects result in other serious health issues, such as cardiac hypertrophy, diastolic dysfunction, and decreased aortic compliance, which are all independent predictors of cardiovascular risk.

Yet, there is a higher prevalence of such diseases, found in people who are overweight, than risk factors for other health problems.

Obesity refers to the excess amount of adipose tissue in the body and is now measured by the body mass index (BMI). This refers to body fat in relation to lean body mass, and anything from 25 to 29.9 kilograms per square meter defines an individual as being overweight, with obesity being calculated as a BMI of ≥30 kilograms per square meter. BMI is the adult's weight in kilograms divided by the square of his or her height and is closely correlated with total body fat content. Abdominal obesity is defined as a waist circumference of >102 centimeters (40 inches) in men and >88 centimeters (35 inches) in women and is much easier to identify visually.

But the problems relating to excess weight and obesity are far more complex than simply reducing an accumulation of fatty tissue, because obesity can influence the water balance or fluid distribution in the body, which makes the loss of such fat more difficult.

This imbalance is involved with blood pressure, osmotic pressure, inflammation, venous system problems, and the body's temperature hormone system.

Because so many factors are involved, and a state of obesity is already related to many systemic imbalances within the body, many people find that weight loss simply does not happen as an outcome of participating in exercise and adjusting the diet. Most treatments and solutions recommended for obesity emphasize increased energy usage and decreased calorie intake, but we can expand this view by examining the relationships between organic systems.

In my personal opinion, we focus on medical complications arising from obesity and being overweight, but these are secondary issues or, if you will, side effects. The obesity itself is a medical condition irrespective of any problems that may or may not have arisen, and it needs to be monitored, cured, and treated as a chronic disorder.

Acupuncture is used not only for a wide variety of health conditions, but also simply to maintain optimal health. When used in patients suffering from symptoms such as bloating and chronic back and arthritic pain, particularly where digestive motility is also affected, it can help to relieve symptoms subjectively. This, in itself, usually assists in increasing the motivation and mobility of many patients.

For those who have embarked on a diet and exercise program but find that they are struggling to lose weight, or have even gained weight, it may be considered that other health issues, such as hormonal dysfunction, muscle dystrophy due to disuse, or a clinical history of trauma, are causing the problems they encounter. The six body types treatment is not aimed at curing or treating the diagnosed disease, but it can assist in identifying the structural and functional parts affected. By restoring the body balance, it may also assist in restoring internal organ function indirectly and support any weight loss program.

4

Body Posture and Homeostasis

We have familiarized ourselves with the specialty and specialization of parts of the whole. Digging the hole deeper, we can see the sky through the hole, but not in its entirety. The body is more than the gathering of the parts, and the connectedness of human structure and function is the big picture in understanding our body.

Body posture is the entire structure of the human state, the integration of the bones, muscles, nerves, and blood vessels, and homeostasis explains how the normal interaction between structure and function is adjusted and maintained. This integration of structural information and functional concept is based on body anatomy and physiology.

How can we determine the connection between the body structure and homeostasis? A good departure point would be to think about the cycle of life. Body organs and structures gradually grow until maturity, and body organ functions develop at the same time. At the point of maturity, in the early 20s, healthy adult body structures and functions are fully matured and developed. The function of homeostasis is to maintain this peak status. Following this period, the body repair system is not as effective and the body structure is damaged or changed through atrophy. Because of structural atrophy, the body's physiologic functions decrease. During these periods, the body changes externally and internally; the body's external structure will change while the internal hormonal levels are raised or decreased. The structural change of the body is synched to the internal physiologic changes.

When we think about the life cycle of the human body, we note that the body organ functions have been adapted and transformed to change the body structure (growing and aging) constantly during the entire life span. Even though organ transplant surgeries, childbirth complications, and hormonal medications bring about substantial changes in the body, the body function shows miraculous adaptation and alteration over time.

In the 1800s, a famous French physiologist, Claude Bernard, suggested that the internal environment of the animal's body consists of tissue fluid that bathes the cells. He concluded that the relative stability of the internal environment allows animals to live in the external, often unstable environment.

Later, American physiologist Walter Cannon introduced the term *homeostasis*. Homeostasis is the dynamic yet stable condition of internal environment regardless of external environment. All organ systems contribute to homeostasis, which includes blood glucose level stability in the liver, pH regulation in the kidneys, and body temperature regulation in hormonal and nervous systems. Once homeostasis stabilizes the system, the body's metabolism is able to function efficiently.

In the 1980s, the concept of allostasis was proposed by Sterling and Eyer to describe an additional process of reestablishing homeostasis. According to the allostasis theory, the primary difference between homeostasis and allostasis is that the principle of homeostasis assumes that an organism attempts to maintain internal stability, while the theory of allostasis states that the organism attempts to regulate its internal systems in the way that is most adaptive to the current situation, based on the organism's prior experiences. The principles of allostasis claim that stability is less important than adaptability and that internal systems are not designed to be perfectly stable.

I think that the term *balance* in organisms is not to be compared to the absolute, measuring seesaw balance, but might be more like the helix backbone of the DNA strand's spiral motion in space. The DNA is a double-helix structure linked by bases, like the rungs on a twisted ladder. There are four bases of paired RNA, and two polynucleotide chains running in opposite directions. The two DNA strands wind around the helix axis like the railing of a spiral staircase.

Its structural form is composed of substances, directions, periods, directivity, and latent ability.

CHINESE MEDICINE, BALANCE, AND HOMEOSTASIS

In traditional Chinese medicine (TCM), balancing is one of the most popular terms with regard to pathogenic diagnosis and treatments. The theory of yin and yang, presented in the Yin and Zhou dynasty (16–22 B.C.), is applied to the field of medicine and guided clinical work up to the present. It emphasizes the balancing and interrelationship between yin and yang. Since yin and yang explains phenomena, the Qi basic motion theory was added to present the dynamic physical principles.

Dynamic motion is the opposition between yin and yang, which can generate the force of all change and development. Yin and yang are constantly in a stage of balance while they consume and transform each other, such as in "yang to the yin, yin to the yang."

This philosophy and fundamental theory is applied to traditional Chinese medicine and includes diagnosis, physiology, pathology, treatment plan, treatment modalities, and so forth. Even within the arena of anatomy and physiology, yin and yang explains body structures and organ systems according to specific characteristics and functions. According to the ancient TCM book *Simple Question* in Chapter 5, "Yang transforms Qi, Yin transforms the structure." For example, the physiologic phenomenon corresponds to the yang aspect, and the anatomical structure corresponds to the yin. In yin and yang theory, the combination of the two looks like a coin with heads and tails, or a wheel with a front and rear. When Qi is added, the coin or wheel is ready to roll along.

WU XING

Within yin and yang and Qi theory, Wu Xing is a fundamental theory in traditional Chinese medicine that expresses the natural phenomenon metaphorically. A further important theory, 五行 (the five phasic cycle), has been misinterpreted as the five-element theory. The 五行 Wu Xing does not explain the static absolute elements, but the changes of natural processes in certain phases of cycle and movement.

In each phase of a cycle, a particular element is applied to corresponding organs, characteristics, functions, qualities, colors, and most natural items that need to be explained or identified. The five movements have sequential reactions, such as promoting, controlling, bullying, and insulting, while they are arranged in order according to their qualities based on water, wood, fire, earth, and metal qualities. Sometimes earth is arranged at the center of the phasic explanation.

I like to imagine a line graph with an x and y axis, with earth at the center, fire at the top of the y, and water at the bottom of the y axis. Wood is on the far right of the x, and metal is on the far left of the x. Fire (top of y) is the yang quality, water (bottom of y) is the yin quality. Wood (far right of x) is active, while metal (far left of x) is less active.

The shape of the sphere is the result of formation with all the interactions, mutual interrelationships, and cyclic movements in a specific time and space. Each phase corresponds to organs, characters, functions, qualities, or colors. The five phases move in sequential order: wood, fire, earth, metal, and water.

Furthermore, each phase has functional interactions, such as interpromoting, interacting, overacting, and counteracting, which constantly adjust the balance of power. With yin and yang, Wu Xing is important for explaining the homeostasis cyclic phenomenon in TCM. This philosophy and foundation are applied to various aspects of traditional Chinese medicine, such as diagnosis, physiology, pathology, treatment plan, and treatment modalities. In view of balance, there are two dimensions, three dimensions, and a cyclic sphere.

TCM LIFE CYCLES

There are many interpretations of the cyclic phenomenon in TCM theories, and the TCM life cycles are divided by gender. While the woman's cycle is seven years, the man's cycle is eight years, and both are determined by major hormonal changes. It has been observed and described that the body's physical changes occur as a result of the internal hormonal system changes.

At seven years old, a girl's kidney energy is abundant and her milk teeth are replaced by permanent teeth. Her hair also grows longer and stronger. At the age of 14, her first menstruation starts when the Ren and Chong meridian are flourishing and abundant, and she can conceive at this point. At 21 years old, her kidney energy has reached its peak so her wisdom teeth emerge. Her height and body structure have reached their peak. At 28 years old, her tendons and bones are stronger and her hair growth at it strongest. The body condition is strong and flourishing. At the age of 35, her condition starts to decline, especially from the Yang Ming channel, which is related to the digestive system. The complexion starts to fade and she begins to lose hair. At the age of 42, her face is darker and her hair begins to turn gray. The three yang channels become weaker. At 49 years old, the Ren and Chong meridian is empty and depleted and menstruation ceases. She is no longer able to conceive.

The life cycle of a man is different. At eight years old, his body's kidney energy is abundant, and his hair and teeth grow. At the age of 16, his kidney energy is more abundant and kidney essence will transform into sperm. At the age of 24, the kidney energy is at its peak and his growth is at its peak. The wisdom teeth emerge and tendons and bones are strong. At 32 years old, his tendons and bones are at their strongest, and muscles are full and strong. At the age of 40, the kidneys start to weaken, he experiences hair loss, and the teeth loosen. At 48 years old, his yang energy of body is depleted from the upper body and his face will start to darken, while his hair changes to gray. At the age of 56, the liver energy weakens, sperm begins to dry up, and the kidneys become weak. His overall body energy is weak and grows old. At the age of 64, the hair and teeth are gone.

Biological Rhythms

A biological rhythm is any cyclic change in the level of a bodily chemical or function. Two major factors influence the internal and external system. Endogenous rhythm is controlled by the internal biological clock and affects aspects such as the body temperature cycle and the eating digestion cycle. Exogenous rhythm is controlled by synchronizing internal cycles with external stimuli such as seasonal weather changes and day and night. These stimuli are called *zeitgebers*, a term first used by Jürgen Aschoff, one of the founders of the field of chronobiology. A zeitgeber is any external or environmental stimulus that affects the organism's biological rhythms in relation to the earth's 24-hour light–dark cycle and 12-month cycle.

Several different terms indicate period and time. The circadian rhythms are endogenously generated rhythms with a period close to 24 hours. Diurnal rhythms are synchronized with the day–night cycle. Ultradian rhythms are much shorter periodic cycles. For example, the three-meal cycle is included in ultradian rhythms. Infradian rhythms are cycles of more than 24 hours, such as the menstrual cycle.

The circulatory cycle is important for body function. It includes heartbeat rhythm, the inhale and exhale cycle, and blood vessel pressure diastole–systole volume wave rhythms. The internal body organs constantly move in their own rhythmical motion according to certain biomechanical movements.

Kidney and Kidney Essence

The rhythm and beat of our heart can be heard in our earliest life, even before we are born. The fetus can feel the heartbeat, breathing rhythms, and voice of its mother in the womb. We have five senses: hearing, sight, smell, taste, and touch. Of these senses, the first experienced may be hearing the outside world.

Traditional Chinese medical theory addresses the relationship between the kidney and the ear. It emphasizes that the kidney has the prenatal and postnatal essences for growth and development. According to the Neijing Suwen, "The kidney Qi communicates with the ears; if the kidney functions properly, the ears can distinguish the five essential sounds." In fact, the ear and the kidney develop around the fifth to eighth week of pregnancy. The kidney and the cochlea of the inner ear have some very similar membranes that are held together with a substance called collagen. These membranes are similar in function and in structure, and in both cases, these membranes help maintain the chemical balance of the fluids of the kidney and the inner ear. Because of their similar molecular structure, they can be damaged by the same medications or toxic substances, such as an overdose of diuretics.

These periodic life cycles are determined by the kidney essence, the organic substance in TCM. This essence forms the basis of growing, reproducing, developing, and aging. The kidney holds the essence, but it is also circulated throughout the body, particularly in the eight extraordinary vessels that are treated in cases of abnormal functioning, that is, homeostatic imbalances.

These eight extraordinary vessels are very important in type S of the six body types because the effects of the chronic stage of hormonal imbalance can be expressed by the channel system, which can then be effected on body structure as deformed and reformed. I explain more about eight extraordinary vessels in detail later in this chapter.

EIGHT PRINCIPLES: PATTERN OF BODY BALANCE IDENTIFICATION

In traditional Chinese medicine, all symptoms of diseases are based on the theory of eight principles. There are several differential identification theories of disorder by quality of diseases, periodic states, and progress of diseases and the level of body. The four levels theory comprises the Wei (defensive), Qi level, Ying (nutritive), and Xue (blood) stages according to the progress of diseases. Another theory related to progress of disorder is the six stages, which was proposed by Zhang Zhongjing in the *Shang Han Lun* (translated as "On Cold Damage") from about 220 A.D., or about 1700 years ago. The six stages are identified by acupuncture meridian names and explain the progress of external pathogens penetrating into the body.

The eight-principle pattern identification is formulated with four pairs of fundamental qualities of a disease. These pairs are exterior and interior, hot and cold, vacuity and repletion, and yin and yang. The opposition of the pairs represented in the eight principles theory is for assessing the imbalance of body state.

Exterior versus Interior Identification

The exterior syndrome affects skin, hair, muscular interstices, and superficial parts of meridians and collaterals. The interior syndrome affects the visceral, Qi, blood, and bone marrow. If the exterior and interior parts are close enough to communicate, the body looks bright, healthy, and younger. If not, dark complexion, wrinkles, stretch marks, and unhealthy changes take place.

The pathogenic identifications, the exterior patterns, are the primary stage of an invasion of the six pathogenic factors into the body through the skin, mouth, and nose. It is marked by a sudden onset, a short duration, and a shallow location. The interior patterns are dysfunctions of the organs and imbalance between Qi and blood. This

40 • *Body Reshaping through Muscle and Skin Meridian Therapy*

is due to impairment of internal organs through intrinsic pathogens such as emotional upsets, imbalanced diet, and irregular daily lifestyle.

Hot and Cold Identifications

In hot and cold identifications, heat syndrome describes the possible symptoms and signs as fever, aversion to heat with preference for cold, red complexion or flushed cheeks, thirst with preference for cold drinks, restlessness, insomnia, yellow and sticky sputum, vomiting blood and epistaxis, scanty brown urine, dry feces, red tongue with scanty moisture, and rapid pulse. This group of symptoms and signs suggest that the internal or external body has inflammation or infection as well as hyperactive body systems.

The cold syndrome presents with the following symptoms and signs: aversion to cold or intolerance of cold with preference for warmth, cold limbs and huddling up in sleep, pale complexion, moist mouth without thirst, thin sputum, clear and profuse urine, loose stool, pale moist tongue with white, slippery coating, and slow or tense pulse. These cold patterns are related to body thermoregulation impairment, blood circulation, or sedentary lifestyle.

Vacuity (Deficiency) and Repletion (Excess) Identification

For vacuity and repletion patterns, the etiologies are important. The vacuity patterns are as follows:

- Congenital Qi deficiency: Genetic factors
- Insufficient production of Qi and blood due to malnutrition: Nutritional imbalance, poor diet habit

- Impairment of organ Qi and blood due to emotional factors, stress, overwork, too much exercise, and sleep disorders
- Exhaustion of kidney essence due to excessive sexual intercourse
- Impairment of healthy Qi due to chronic disease: After hospitalization or during the postpartum period

For the repletion pattern, there are two different body conditions: healthy immune system and organ function weakness. A healthy, strong immune system is able to carry out the immune defense processes, such as fever and acute inflammations, and to sound the alarm when there an invasion of pathogenic factors into the body. The other condition is the dysfunction of organs leading to the accumulation of phlegm, fluids, dampness, and blood stagnation in the body.

Yin and Yang Identification

Yin and yang integrate all aspects classified under generalizing syndrome patterns, which includes the three pairs of eight theory. The pattern of yin syndrome develops slowly in both onset and recovery, whereas the yang pattern develops rapidly in both onset and recovery. Within the eight extraordinary channels system, these eight principles of pattern identification are used to diagnose and assess the stage of patients in my clinic.

HOMEOSTASIS

We now understand that the adaption, periodic changing, developing cells and organs, and state of pulling and pushing against the periodic axis are the homeostasis. Homeostasis has three communication systems, which include the organs, organ control system, and negative loop. When one of these systems loses efficiency, the body enters the stage of illness, and gradually other organ systems become affected. Homeostasis dysfunction means that the body is in a state of disorder and disease.

Several factors cause homeostatic dysfunction, such as hormones, behavior, external trauma, and internal system dysfunctions. Once body homeostatic dysfunctions have occurred, we feel subjectively hot or cold, fullness or emptiness, thirsty or heavy, urgency or lazy, and sweet or salty food cravings. Because the body aims to balance body function, homeostasis will generate behavior motivation.

For this reason, hormonal therapy may be advised by practitioners for hormonal imbalance disorder, such as diabetes mellitus and hypertension. The single treatment method does not deliver satisfactory results. In the case of patients who have experienced weight gain or body structure change due to hormonal dysfunction, the practitioner needs to assess the entire spectrum of the lifestyle, behavior, habits, and other environmental factors of the patient in order to prepare a long-term treatment plan. Similar to musculoskeletal adaptations, the internal organs and soft tissues adapt and change their structures and functions within the survival ranges. The observation of habit and behavior is important for understanding the pathologic mechanism.

Water and Salt Intake and Body Fluid Homeostasis

Human body tissues depend on the nutrients delivered by circulating blood to support the cellular metabolism and get rid of waste products from the metabolites. Every cell in the body is connected to the watery body matrix. Water is the largest part of the body and contributes about 55%–65% of normal body weight. The body attempts to maintain an adequate amount of water and regulates the volume through osmotic homeostasis and volume homeostasis.

Body fluids in the blood vessels are moved by osmotic and hydrostatic pressure. The protein and sodium in blood vessels attract cellular fluids. If the blood protein level decreases due to malnutrition or other disorder, the fluids remain in the cell membrane, which leads to edema.

There are four conditions that imbalance water homeostasis: hypovolemia, hypervolemia, dehydration, and overhydration. Hemorrhage or blood loss due to trauma affects the volume of blood and body fluids and results in hypovolemia. Sweating after vigorous exercise causes a loss of body fluids through the skin, and this can lead to the body becoming dehydrated. Even the administering of intravenous fluids causes plasma volume to increase rapidly, and if the oncotic pressure exchange has not occurred, this condition results in hypervolemia. Drinking too much water can dilute the plasma in the blood vessels, and osmolarity then decreases and results in overhydration. However, overhydration does not usually occur in healthy individuals. Overhydration may occur in those with faulty kidney function and who, especially, excrete excessive amounts of urine.

Although the primary role of the kidneys is concerned with osmotic homeostasis, the skin and lungs also play a role in the process of osmoregulation. Water and electrolytes are lost through sweat glands in the skin, while small amounts of water evaporate from the lungs. The kidneys maintain osmotic regulation and blood pressure in the body and are involved in the production of hormones.

The adrenal medulla releases epinephrine and norepinephrine, which are the flight and fight hormones related to stress. During stress, the body instantly prepares against danger with great energy. Epinephrine and norepinephrine also decrease kidney function temporarily by vasoconstriction. Other hormones involved in osmoregulation include renin, angiotensin, aldosterone, and antidiuretic hormone (ADH).

Homeostatic regulation is not just controlled by the central hormonal system, but is also assisted by the promotion of the mechanism intrinsic to the physiology of body fluids, such as the cardiovascular system. The behavior motivations to regulate water balance within the body are expressed by thirst and craving salty food. Thirst, and the water intake it provokes, is a much more rapid and less limited response to dehydration than antidiuresis. The feeling of thirst is subjectively described by the burning, bitter, and bad taste in the mouth. Thirst may be defined as a strong motivation to seek, obtain, and consume water in response to deficits in body fluids. Stress and anxiety can sometimes be triggers to drink water, because sudden stress hormones from the kidney have an effect on vasoconstrictions.

In TCM, taste is linked to the disharmony in corresponding organ systems, such as a sour taste for liver disharmony, a bitter taste for the heart system, a sweet taste for spleen deficiency, a pungent taste for lungs, and a salty taste for kidney deficiency. These references are also used in the formulation of herbal medicine. For example, if a patient has cold symptoms, the pungent or spicy quality of herbs is used in the formula,

because the spicy quality stimulates the body's chemical reaction of pain sensation and warms the nerve fibers, and the body responds with the physical reactions of heat, including vasodilation and sweating. Severe thirst occurs when loss of blood or hypovolemic symptoms are first detected by the blood vessel stretch receptors in the large veins entering the right atrium of the heart.

Furthermore, food plays an important role in regulating and balancing the body fluids. Balanced meals provide enough iron and protein in the blood vessels to maintain the blood volume and collect the fluids from within the interstitial space. In instances of craving too much salt, it is recommended that the body system be examined to determine the cause. However, malnutrition and consuming too little salt also affect the body fluids balancing system. Since the body's regulation system adapts gradually to the environment and behavior, knowing and self-tracking your physical condition is important to prevent disease, instead of following the latest trend.

One's drinking habit is not always driven by thirst, but I believe that social, neurological, and psychological factors can influence behavior changes. The information from commercial campaigns has a huge influence on individuals. For example, one of my patients stopped drinking coffee and switched to green tea because she believed that her friend experienced better health by cutting down on caffeine, even though she had indigestion and was uncomfortable when she drank green tea. Coffee and green tea both contain caffeine.

Green tea contains polyphenols, which may prevent inflammation and swelling and protect cartilage between the bones, and it has antiviral effects. However, in Chinese food theory of taste and functions, the coffee has a warmer quality than the green tea, which means the colder quality can make the digestive system sluggish, depending on the conditions, especially with regard to absorption. Furthermore, green tea is believed to have diuretic effects. Since green tea is known as the diet tea for this reason, green tea is as a weight loss supplement. Sudden diet changes and diuretic methods can temporarily result in weight loss and feeling light, but the body fluids regulation system is adjusted when the body organ and hormone effectors are stable.

Alcohol also affects body fluids regulation; it inhibits secretion of ADH, increases urine output, leads to dehydration, slows the metabolism as it is a central nervous system (CNS) depressant, stimulates insulin secretion, and lowers blood sugar levels.

IMMUNE FUNCTION AND THERMOREGULATION

Humans normally regulate body (core) temperature at about 37°C (98.6°F), and fluctuations within the narrow range of 35°C–41°C (95°F–105.8°F) can be tolerated by healthy individuals; core temperatures outside this range can induce morbidity and mortality.

Heat exhaustion is defined as a syndrome of hyperthermia; the body temperature escalates beyond normal to ≤40°C (104°F) and is a debilitation that occurs during or immediately after exertion in the heat, accompanied by headache. It results in insufficient cardiac output, frequently accompanied by sweaty, hot skin, dehydration, and collapse.

Heat injury is a moderate to severe illness characterized by evidence of damage to organs, such as liver, kidney, digestive system, and tissues, without sufficient neurologic symptoms to be diagnosed as heat stroke. It is usually associated with body temperatures above 40°C (104°F).

Heatstroke is a severe illness characterized by profound mental status changes with high body temperatures, usually, but not always, higher than 40°C (104°F).

When the body temperature fluctuates, body homeostatic thermoregulation is taking place. When the temperature is elevated, skin eccrine sweat glands secrete body fluids for evaporating and cooling the skin, and arteriolar vasodilation allows for heat loss through conduction and convection. On the other hand, if the body temperature is too low, the skin pores close to prevent heat loss and vasoconstriction takes place, which makes the skin pale and numb in severe cases. The hypothalamus sends a signal to the muscles and they shiver, which generates heat. Another form of thermogenesis takes place through the sympathetic outflow to brown fat cells, brown adipose tissue (BAT), which is abundant in newborn babies and hibernating animals. Brown fat cells are located on the upper chest or in the neck skin and muscle area exposed to the external environment.

The skin has an important role in regulating body temperature as a part of homeostatic function, as well as an active immune organ. Fever is an immune response that raises the body temperature and, in so doing, protects the body from infection and injury. This action is the hypothalamus's change of the thermostat point for the body defense mechanism, unlike hyperthermia. With cold symptoms, body aches, indigestion, and body stuffiness accompany the raised temperature because the peripheral blood moves toward the internal body for reducing heat loss and generating heat from muscles contracting and shivering. Once the pathogenic factors are cleared and the body thermostat is reset to the normal level, the blood moves to the skin and clears the heat through the skin via sweat. If a healthy individual has a viral or bacterial infection and a fever, the symptoms are cleared after several days and fever is eradicated without any medication. However, some people cannot, or are less able to, generate a fever.

The substances responsible for fever are the pyrogens, such as lymphocytes and neutrophils. Lymphocytes are predominantly produced in the presence of a viral infection, and neutrophils in a bacterial infection. These pyrogens act on the hypothalamus to change the thermostat and allow fever. When a person cannot produce a fever at the appropriate time, we can assume several possibilities. First, the thermoregulatory center has been disturbed; second, there are insufficient endogenous pyrogens; and third, the sensitivity of the pyrogens is weak. Impaired immune responses also can cause frequent infection and inflammation, which results in reduced fever response. The body has an innate immune system that provides immediate defense against infection. The innate immune system includes phagocytosis, inflammation, acid secretions of the stomach, digestive enzymes, and skin.

Frequently recurring cold symptoms are related to immune deficiency. Interestingly, immune deficiency in children and adolescents is connected to adult obesity. Since the skin and digestive system play the most important roles in immune and thermoregulation, childhood skin conditions and digestive system issues can be managed and protected from pathogenic factors.

The skin's exposure to cold can cause the peripheral vasoconstriction to reduce heat transfer between the body's core and skin and subcutaneous area. Repeated exposure to the cold can elicit muscle contraction, which prevents the flow of peripheral blood to the skin and shell. This vasoconstriction results in a thickening and separates the shell from underlying muscles. Clinical observation often finds cases of skin and muscle-isolated conditions in chronic muscle tension and chronic stress patients.

In TCM, a famous clinical book, *Shang Han Lun*, known in English as the *Treatise on Cold Damage Disorders* or the *Treatise on Cold Injury*, is a Chinese medical treatise compiled by Zhang Zhong Jing (张仲景) at the end of the Han dynasty. This book clearly describes the six channels as a basis for diagnosis and explains the etiology and pathological development of externally contracted febrile disease. The periodic observations explain the cold, temperature, thermoregulation, and immune reaction with a summary of disease patterns, formulae, and treatment principles. For example, the first stage of febrile disease, it explains, includes the symptoms of fever, sweat, and the patient's energy level. Each formula is then prescribed according to the symptoms. If the patient has too much vasoconstriction, then prescribe the quality of vasodilation for inducing sweat and assist the migration of immune cells. If a patient has enterovirus symptoms, prescribed the spicy and sour quality formula for inducing digestive enzymes and acid secretions in the stomach.

Respiratory System and Homeostasis

Each cell of the body is constantly bathed in the fluid environment that brings and supplies the oxygen and removes the carbon dioxide from metabolic by-products. The homeostatic balance of the body depends on the respiratory function because the mitochondria in each cell require the oxygen for their energy conversion, while at the same time the energy conversion produces waste products, including carbon dioxide, that need to be discarded through the gas exchange system. Respiratory homeostasis is closely related to cellular homeostasis.

Living includes the ability to move internally and externally, and when physical activities increase, cellular respiration increases and generates more carbon dioxide. Once the carbon dioxide level is increased in blood vessels, the sense detector stimulates the medulla oblongata to drive heart and breathing muscles. The medulla oblongata stimulates an increased heart rate to bring the carbon dioxide from the blood vessel to the lungs more rapidly. It also stimulates the breathing muscles to force the breathing out of carbon dioxide more rapidly from the body. Then the level of carbon dioxide is returned to the normal range. This is a simplified loop for the respiratory balance system.

The breathing, respiratory homeostatic system has many mechanisms involved interdependently, such as the cardiovascular system, nervous system, skeletal muscles, immune system, and pH homeostasis. During vigorous exercise, the heart rate increases, and breathing is forced by the chest and abdominal muscles known as respiratory muscles. These muscles help to inhale and exhale, and move the thoracic cavity and abdominal cavity by expansion and contraction.

On the other hand, if the individual has inhaled too much and did not breathe out sufficiently, whether due to emotional distress, physical exertion, or panic attack, a brown bag is used as a breathing tool. The carbon dioxide breathed out into the brown bag is inhaled to balance the blood oxygen and carbon dioxide levels.

There are two functional respiratory systems, internal and external. The internal respiratory system is the gas exchange in the systemic blood capillaries and cellular respiration. The external respiratory system is the pulmonary ventilation (breathing) and gas exchange in the pulmonary capillaries of the lungs. The important thing is that blood carries the gas and transports it to each cell in body. In other words, while the blood transports respiratory gases to the cell, pulmonary ventilation and external respiration are occurring in the respiratory system, and transport and internal respiration are involved in the circulatory system. Thus, respiratory regulation is not concerned only with the breathing function. It is also part of the respiratory and circulatory systems.

This is another important concept to understand regarding Chinese medicinal Qi circulation in the 12 meridian theories for acupuncture treatment. The basic concept of the meridian is that it is responsible for the circulation of Qi and blood distributed both interiorly and exteriorly across the body. The meridians and collaterals have extensive coverage in contents. Chapters 1 and 47 of *Miraculous Pivot*, the classic ancient Chinese acupuncture book, state that the acupuncture treatment must aim at regulating the flow of Qi. The meridians and collaterals transport blood and Qi to adjust yin and yang, nourish tendons and bones, and improve joint functions.

Blood pH and Homeostasis

pH is the acronym for potential hydrogen, and it is the degree of concentration of hydrogen ions in a substance or solution, the range being from 0 to 14. The optimal pH environment helps enzyme reactions in the body. Each enzyme depends on the shape matching with each substrate. The protein enzyme can be deformed if pH levels are not appropriate. Each enzyme reacts at a different range of pH level.

Body pH level is slightly alkaline except in the stomach. However, pH level is the most critical to blood, which maintains the range between 7.35 and 7.45, strictly. If the blood pH is under 7.35, it becomes acidic. This happens because of the by-products released during metabolism, such as carbon dioxide (CO_2), sulfuric acid, and lactic acid. Especially, carbon dioxide is carried in the blood as hydrogen carbonate ions (bicarbonate), which leads to the formation of hydrogen ions in red blood cells. Hydrogen ions combine with hemoglobin, the iron-containing oxygen-transport metalloproteinase in the red blood cells. They compete with oxygen for space on the hemoglobin if there is too much carbon dioxide in the blood, and this can reduce oxygen transport. The carbon dioxide also combines directly with hemoglobin to form carbaminohemoglobin. This molecule has a lower affinity for oxygen than normal hemoglobin. Excess carbon dioxide can also cause respiratory acidosis. Acidosis means that the hydrogen ions are increased (pH is decreased).

The blood may also become acidic in patients suffering from emphysema, asthma, bronchitis, pneumonia, and pulmonary edema. In these cases, carbon dioxide increases in the blood since it cannot effectively diffuse out of the lungs. When respiratory acidosis occurs, the signs and symptoms that may be seen include headaches, confusion, fatigue, muscle weakness,

shortness of breath, tremors, and sleepiness. Chronic respiratory acidosis also may be secondary to obesity hypoventilation syndrome and neuromuscular disorders, such as amyotrophic lateral sclerosis. In healthy individuals, there are several buffering systems in the body, such as the carbonic acid–bicarbonate buffer system, the protein buffer system, and the phosphate buffer system. The kidney also eliminates hydrogen ions.

Metabolic excretion occurs in the lungs as respiration as well as in the kidneys as renal nitrogen metabolism. When the kidneys are not excreting enough acid from the body, metabolic acidosis results from increased by-products from metabolism. Renal acidosis is associated with an accumulation of urea and creatinine, as well as metabolic acid residues of protein catabolism. One of the metabolic by-products is urea (nitrogen-containing compounds), which is produced in the liver from the breakdown of excess amino acids. This urea is transported by blood to the kidney, where it is excreted as urine. The symptoms of metabolic acidosis vary. They may include headaches, palpitations, anxiety, nausea, vomiting, weight gain, joint pain, rapid breathing, and muscle weakness.

The health benefits of regular exercise and movement have been emphasized for many different reasons. Especially, exercise and body movements can help breathing, blood circulation, and excretion to maintain a healthy body. Blood pH homeostasis is related to excretion and expirations. For this reason, exercise is recommended by health practitioners.

The health benefits of regular exercise include breathing that is more productive, increased blood circulation, and proper excretion.

Bone (Calcium and Phosphate) Homeostasis

Since the blood pH homeostasis aspect is more an excretory function, the calcium homeostasis is more related to the digestive system. Calcium and phosphate homeostasis is mainly linked to the digestive, endocrine, renal, and circulation systems.

Calcium and phosphate (bone) homeostasis is regulated by the digestive system, the hormonal system, the skeletal system, and the kidneys. Most calcium and phosphate are absorbed in the gut, especially in the small intestine, as nutrients, and about 99% of calcium is stored in the bones, which plays an important role for regulating blood calcium level. When blood calcium levels decrease, the stored calcium in the bone moves to the blood. Even though intercellular calcium is small in amount, it has important functions, such as contraction, metabolism, excitability, secretion, transcription, immune responses, fertilization, and development. An important function of calcium is its buffering systemic function for respiratory homeostasis.

A deficiency of blood calcium is called hypocalcemia, and an excess of blood calcium is called hypercalcemia. The symptoms of hypercalcemia are bone pain, kidney stones, and gastrointestinal problems such as indigestion, nausea, vomiting, constipation, muscle weakness, arrhythmia, bradycardia, and depression. The symptoms of hypocalcemia are muscle spasm, anxiety, tetany, heart failure, and diarrhea. Since calcium and phosphate absorption depends on the digestive system, the bone condition osteoporosis may be controlled by maintaining a healthy gut system.

Research has repeatedly shown the relationship among age, nutrition, and bone density. The primary cause of osteoporosis is increasing age, especially in women. Most women reach their maximum bone density by the age of 35, whereas most men reach their maximum bone density by age 40. After reaching peak bone density, the bone mass is maintained through a process involving the breakdown of cells and re-forming (remodeling) of bone. As one becomes older, however, the bones break down more quickly than they re-form.

Several factors affect calcium absorption in the gut system. The positive absorption increasing factors are vitamin D and ingestion with alkali. However, overuse of nutritional supplements may bring the serious health problem known as milk–alkali syndrome, which is due to taking calcium and alkali at the same time. Dietary supplements should never be taken without consultation.

The factors that decrease absorption of calcium in the gut include high vegetable fiber, high fat content, corticosteroid treatment, estrogen deficiency, gastrectomy, intestinal malabsorption syndrome, diabetes mellitus, and renal failure. In my clinical experience, patients who have osteoporosis symptoms have more factors related to their digestive system than to age or their eating habits. This is especially true in instances of lower abdominal area restriction, such as scar tissue from surgery, and a history of gynecological complications.

UNDERSTANDING BODY HOMEOSTASIS AND METABOLISM

Metabolism is the chemical reactions that maintain the body in areas of growth, reproduction, and response to the environment.

Every cell in the body maintains the operation of its metabolic pathways, that is, anabolic and catabolic pathways. You are what you eat, as you are structured by the food you consume. Once the food passes through the digestive system, the metabolic process occurs. Catabolic pathways are needed to convert energy, and anabolic pathways are required to build and form the structure and functional parts of the cells.

The energy metabolic system is integrated with the gastrointestinal, hepatic, urinary, respiratory, nervous, and endocrine systems, as well as skeletal muscles, adipose tissue, and the reproductive and circulatory systems.

The complex food enters the digestive system, which reduces the complex nutrients to simpler forms to allow for their absorption. The circulatory system includes both blood and lymphatic vessels that transport the absorbed nutrients to individual cells for immediate use, or they are carried to the liver, muscle, or other organs for storage. The endocrine system regulates the blood oxygen level needed for phosphorylation, which is the cellular energy cycle system that converts energy to ATP. The by-products from the cellular energy cycle are removed by the urinary system. The skin system is involved in the absorption of vitamin D.

In the human body, four major organic molecules are important: carbohydrates, lipids, proteins, and nucleic acids and related molecules (DNA, RNA, and ATP). Carbohydrate (sugar and starch) is the primary source of chemical energy needed by every cell. It serves a structural role as components of RNA and DNA, which are involved in cell reproduction and protein synthesis.

Lipids are also used to provide energy and serve as vitamins, or they protect vital organs as shock absorbers. They also provide the insulator material for nerves to transmit more rapidly. The steroid hormones composed of lipids regulate many physiological processes.

Proteins have two major roles in the body: structural and functional. Proteins form the structure of the cells, tissues, and organs. Proteins also function as enzymes that carry out chemical reactions in the body.

Even the chemical molecules are differentiated according to their action and character. When we eat food, we can gain the energy, the source of structure, and the connectors between cells and tissues. Sometimes the phrase "following the gut system" may be correct, because these nutrients are needed to replace molecules that have been used up in the body structures and functions. If not provided, the system can become damaged or may not function properly.

There is an interrelationship between homeostasis and metabolism. Homeostasis is needed for metabolism to be maintained efficiently, and metabolism is required for the provision of a stable environment maintained by homeostasis, because the metabolism depends on the chemical reaction of catalyzing enzymes that operate in a consistent body temperature. The metabolic process requires an environment with chemical balance, oxygen level, temperature, and removal of waste products.

Negative feedback is the primary homeostatic mechanism with sensors and the control center. Metabolism is maintained by this feedback loop. The internal body sensor detects changes in temperature or pH level, while the external detector sends the alarm to the hypothalamus in the brain to control the effectors, such as blood vessels, hormones, and the skin. Since all these intricate relationships are required of each balancing loop within the many integrated organ systems involved, the control system is not working well. Since many homeostatic loops are involved, it is hard to fix the entire system by controlling just one loop. For example, diet or exercise cannot treat obesity or hormonal disorder.

Diabetes mellitus and hyper- and hypothyroid problems are well-known disruptions of body metabolism. Obesity and being overweight or underweight are considered significant symptoms.

Stress hyperglycemia is an elevation of the blood glucose level during the intense stress of illness, trauma such as stroke, severe pain, and mental stress. It usually resolves after the stress situation is resolved. However, it must be distinguished from various forms of diabetes mellitus.

The primary causes of most adult diabetes mellitus are insulin resistance and lack of compensatory insulin secretion. Typically, the foundation for insulin resistance is laid at a young age through environmental conditions such as overeating and a sedentary lifestyle. According to current medical opinion, the insulin secretory defects usually start about 10 years before diagnosis of diabetes, and no therapy has been proven to prevent the progressive loss of insulin secretion.

Chronic insulin resistance is associated with other disorders, such as dyslipidemia, central obesity, hypertension, and hyperglycemia. When associated with hypertension, diabetes mellitus is considered a metabolic syndrome that can cause serious disease if not controlled and treated.

In the vague symptoms and signs of metabolic syndrome, the patterns and body shapes are used to classify patients as "apple types," who are described as having a round torso and no waistline, their diaphragm area is congested, and there is an accumulation of fatty tissue.

In clinical observation, the diabetes mellitus patient's upper abdominal area and spinal section, T9–T12, has tension and accumulation. The quality of palpation in this area is different from that in the belly adipose tissues.

Lifestyle and Homeostasis

The best type of exercise is one that the individual will do on a regular basis. Walking is considered one of the best choices because it is easy, safe, and inexpensive. Fast walking can burn as many calories as running, but is less likely to cause injuries than running or jogging. Walking does not require training or special equipment, except for appropriate shoes. In addition, walking is an aerobic and weight-bearing exercise, so it is good for your heart and helps prevent osteoporosis.

The benefits of regular exercise are that it

- Reduces your risk of heart disease, high blood pressure, osteoporosis, diabetes, and obesity
- Keeps joints, tendons, and ligaments flexible, which makes it easier to move around
- Reduces some effects of aging, especially the discomfort of osteoarthritis
- Contributes to mental well-being
- Helps relieve depression, stress, and anxiety
- Increases your energy and endurance
- Helps you sleep better
- Helps you maintain a normal weight by increasing your metabolism (the rate at which you burn calories)

Skeletal and cardiac muscles play key roles in the regulation of systemic energy homeostasis and display remarkable plasticity in their metabolic responses to caloric availability and physical activity. Well-planned, monitored, and not obsessively overtaxing exercise levels are beneficial.

Excessive activity may cause physical damage to tendons, muscles, ligaments, cartilages, bones, and joints. This disrupts the homeostatic balances. For example, young woman athletes, especially those who need to control body weight, may develop eating disorders that can be associated with menstrual dysfunction and subsequent decreased bone mineral density (BMD), or osteoporosis. Disordered eating behavior may impair athletic performance and increase risk of injury. Decreased food intake and fluid and electrolyte imbalance can result in decreased endurance, strength, speed, and ability to concentrate. Because the body initially adapts to these changes, a decrease in performance may not be seen for some time.

Food restriction can result not only in menstrual dysfunction and potentially irreversible bone loss, but also in psychological and other medical complications, including depression, fluid and electrolyte imbalance, and changes in the cardiovascular, endocrine, gastrointestinal, and thermoregulatory systems.

Understanding Structure versus Function

Body homeostasis, balancing of organ function, is regulated by the endocrine system. Hormonal secretion and regulation is mostly related to the hypothalamus. The hypothalamus is located at the brainstem in the diencephalon. It regulates the physiological functions in the body, including growth, metabolism, stress responses, reproduction, osmoregulation, and circadian rhythms. All these functions are involved in maintaining homeostasis according to the environmental conditions.

These systems are related to the sensory and autonomic nervous system, receiving internal and external information, including pain, emotions, and autonomic, endocrine, and somatomotor responses, and the hypothalamus integrates and regulates for proper body functions. Integration of the neural, endocrine, and immune mechanisms to protect the body occurs in the brain.

Once sensory information enters the brain, the responsible motor activities are initiated. These repetitive learning processes form behavior habits and musculoskeletal responses. When we learn about the endocrine systemic disorder, the illustration describes and compares the appearance of the body with an imbalance status such as hypo or hyper.

The shape is not just fat with water distribution in the body, but is also accompanied by certain patterns of symptoms and signs, because most endocrine disorders are integrated and intrinsic in complicated disorders. When the specific diagnosis is made as an endocrine disorder, it has already progressed beyond homeostatic imbalance for a while. The transition stage between health and disorder is critical and must be seen as the turning point for prevention of disease and improvement of health.

Especially in the case of homeostatic imbalance disorder, cooperation between the practitioner and the patient is needed to change habits and behavior. That is my motivation for the development of six body types and their treatment. The educational materials and easily understood information are helpful to lead the patients to better health.

EIGHT EXTRAORDINARY MERIDIANS

While constructing the typology of pathologic body shape, I found that the eight extraordinary channels theory is based on the patterns that result from homeostatic imbalances. The symptoms and signs are very brief and difficult to determine from the ancient book. The term *extraordinary channels* is represented as the abnormal status of channels. According to the function of the eight extraordinary channels, they differ from the 12 main meridians and do not pertain to the Zang organs (kidney, heart, liver, spleen, and lung) and communicate with the Fu organs (urinary bladder, gallbladder, stomach, small intestine, and large intestine). Furthermore, the *Classic of Difficulties* compares the extraordinary channels to reservoirs that are able to absorb excessive Qi and blood from the primary channels in the same way that reservoirs take excess water from canals and ditches during times of heavy rain.

In the Ming dynasty, the study of the eight extraordinary vessels by Li Shi Zhen showed that when the Qi of the channels overflows, it flows into the extraordinary vessels, where it is turned into irrigation, warming the organs internally and irrigating the space between skin and muscle externally. The extraordinary vessels all originate directly or indirectly from the kidneys, and they contain the essence stored in the kidneys.

In certain pathogenic environments, especially shock and stress, the body's regular function of Qi and blood flow is disturbed and the surplus moves to another extraordinary path to protect from outside pathogenic factors and store the surplus. However, when the regular meridian is weak, the surplus is not able to provide what is lacking. It appears that the immune protein migrates to the subcutaneous tissue or lymphatic fatty tissue accumulated in the area.

The classification of patterns of homeostatic imbalance has similar patterns seen by structural changes, such as the buffalo hump of Cushing syndrome, the goiter of thyroid disorder, gastroparesis of diabetes mellitus, and edema of chronic renal failure. Some endocrine disorders are predictive of health risks and can be differentiated by typical body patterns, such as abdominal fat and frequently swollen legs.

I wondered whether there was a possibility that a severe disorder could be prevented if the body structure was changed before the condition worsened, but I would need to understand the mechanism and pattern first. Fortunately, the clue was in the eight extraordinary channel systems that explain the entire body's systemic path, and pathogenic symptoms, signs, and treatment. The eight extraordinary meridians are the largest contributor to the initial idea of six body types.

The eight extraordinary vessels (channels, meridians) include the directing (Ren), governing (Du), penetrating (Chong), girdle (Dai), yin and yang stepping, and yin and yang linking vessels.

The three major channels are the governing (Du channel), directing (Ren), and penetrating (Chong) meridians that start from the lower abdominal area in the space between the kidneys.

Du Channel

The Du channel links all the yang channels at du14, which is located in the depression below the spinous process of the seventh cervical vertebra (Figure 4.1). The Du channel starts from the lower abdomen and emerges on the perineum, then follows the spine upward. The channel goes into the brain and ends on the gum in the mouth. The Du channel is known as the sea of yang channels and helps regulate the Qi of all the yang channels.

Ren Channel

The Ren channel meets all the yin meridians, and it is called the sea of yin channels (Figure 4.2). It rises from the lower abdomen and follows the midline of the body until it winds around the mouth and ascends to the eye. Another branch of the Ren channel rises from the pelvic cavity and ascends along the spine internally.

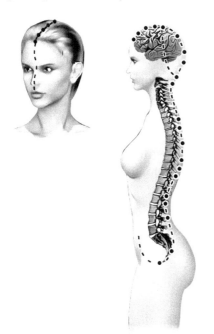

FIGURE 4.1
Du channel.

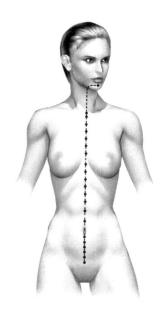

FIGURE 4.2
Ren channel.

Chong Channel

The Chong channel links the stomach and kidney channels and strengthens the link between the Ren from the pelvic cavity and the Du (Figure 4.3). It is known as the sea of blood. The Chong channel ascends and runs parallel with the kidney meridian, communicating with Ren channels in the lower abdominal area. The kidney channel is very closely located on the midline to the xiphoidal process, and then spreads toward the sides of the breast area. The Chong channel ascends through the liver and diaphragm and enters the lung before joining with the heart and pericardium channel. The other branch goes to the lower coccyx to the lumbar spine and enters the kidneys and urinary bladder. The Chong channel also runs downward on the medial side of the thigh and terminates at the medial side of the big toe.

I imagine that the channel path of the Du meridian is associated with the central nervous system, the Ren meridian is

Body Posture and Homeostasis • 53

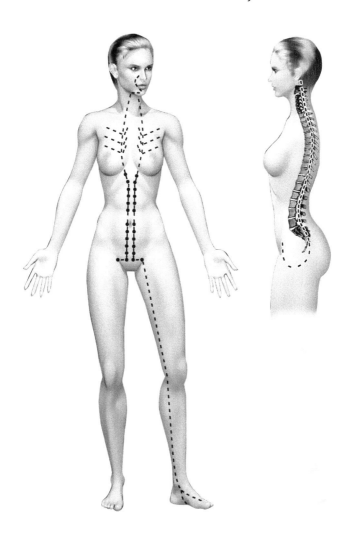

FIGURE 4.3
Chong channel.

associated with the hormonal axis, and the Chong meridian is associated with blood circulation to major organs. They seem like nervous, endocrine, and circulatory systems. Together, the nervous and endocrine systems coordinate functions of all body systems. The nervous system controls homeostasis through nerve impulses conducted along axons of neurons, which results in quick responses. In contrast, the endocrine system releases its hormones into the bloodstream. The circulating blood then delivers hormones to virtually all cells throughout the body. Therefore, hormones work relatively slowly and for longer periods, and they, especially endocrine, are carried by blood vessels, though apocrine and paracrine are not necessarily carried by blood vessels. The Du and Ren channels have their own meridian points, and other meridians share their points with other main meridians.

Following the pathologic description from the classic book, the points of the Du channel are mainly applied to the disorders of the brain and nervous system, that is, mental and emotional disorders. If there is severe illness of the Du channel, the book describes a condition similar to paroxysmal sympathetic hyperactivity.

Paroxysmal sympathetic hyperactivity is a syndrome that causes episodes of increased activity of the sympathetic nervous system. Hyperactivity of the sympathetic nervous system can manifest as increased heart rate, increased respiration, increased blood pressure, diaphoresis, and hyperthermia.

Dai Channel

The Dai channel is also called the belt vessel, as it flows around the lower waistline (Figure 4.4). It is situated below the hypochondriac area at the level of the second lumbar vertebra, turns downward, and encircles the body at the waist like a girdle. The Dai channel binds up all the meridians. If the Dai channel has disorder, a feeling of heaviness of the body, coldness of the back, as if sitting in water, and fullness of the abdomen occur. The Dai channel path is similar to the transverse abdominis muscle that runs within the rib cage, iliac crest, and spine. This muscle is known as the core muscle, along with spinal multipidi muscles. If these muscles are weak, the lumbar spine may curve like "lordosis" and the abdomen will protrude. These muscles help delivery in childbirth. Since this area is circular and is formed primarily by muscles, fascia, ligaments, and soft tissue, the range of motion is different from that of other skeletal muscle areas. The Dai channel should be flexible and loosen with circular motion, such as a Hawaiian hula dance or a Middle Eastern belly dance, the movements of which are most beneficial for getting rid of upper side back area water congestions. I will explain more about the circular motion and the Dai channel in the type S in Chapter 5.

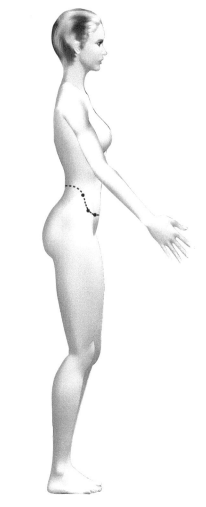

FIGURE 4.4
Dai channel.

Yang and Yin Heel Channels

The Yang heel and Yin heel channels meet each other at the inner canthus (Figures 4.5 and 4.6). Motion regulation of the lower limbs is their joint function, especially ankle joints. The yang heel channel follows the urinary bladder (UB) channel, outer malleolus, and the yin heel channel follows the kidney channel, inner malleolus. These channels relate to movement, and body structure and conditions. Equinus is an example of an ankle problem. If the

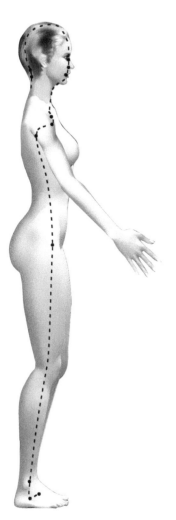

FIGURE 4.5
Yang heel channel.

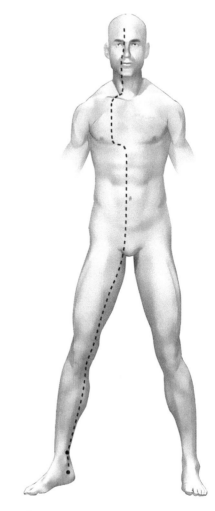

FIGURE 4.6
Yin heel channel.

ankle problem is not remedied, the postural problem associated with equinus leads to a tightening or shortening of the gastrocnemius and soleus, and results in a spinal curvature deformity. This condition causes a hyper extended (flexed) ankle shape when the person lies down in a supine position. If a patient presents with a dorsiflexion when lying down, the symptoms provide clues to the patient's motion history; for example, a tibialis muscle problem indicates excessive walking in the mountains.

YANG AND YIN LINKING CHANNELS

Yang and yin linking vessels regulate the flow of Qi in the yin and yang meridians and help maintain coordination and equilibrium between the yin and yang meridians (Figures 4.7 and 4.8). The yang linking channel connects with all the yang meridians and dominates the exterior of the entire body with all the yang meridians. It has been stated that the

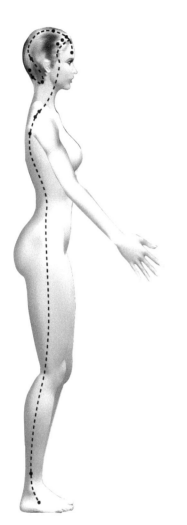
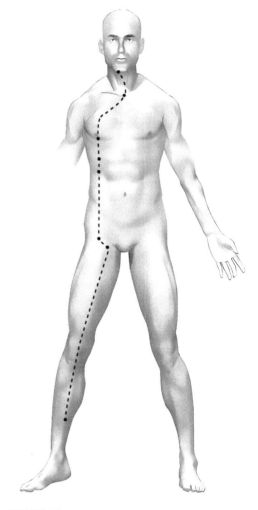

FIGURE 4.7
Yang linking channel.

FIGURE 4.8
Yin linking channel.

exterior of the entire body is Wei Qi. If the yang linking channel has disorder, then the patient may alternately feel hot and cold, be averse to cold, have a fever, and experience backache with sudden swelling. It appears that exterior pathogenic factors such as viruses and bacteria invade the body and disrupt the body thermoregulation and immune systems.

In clinical use, the Dai channel is paired with the yang linking channel. According to the Dai channel disorder description, the sensation of a heavy, waterlogged feeling on the side of the back is mentioned. With regard to the yang linking channel, the hot and cold sensation occurs if the channel has disorder. The yang linking channel is related to the Wei Qi, which is the resistance against exterior pathogenic factors.

The yin linking vessel connects with all yin meridians and dominates the interior of the whole body. If the yin linking vessel has disorder, heart pain, chest pain, fullness and pain of the lateral costal region, and lumbar pain are experienced. The yin linking to the Chong channel can be used in diagnosis by palpation of the area. It is important to pay attention to any palpitations, hard masses, discoloration, and blood vessel shapes.

In my understanding and application of the eight extraordinary channels for diagnosis and treatment, the following rules are devised:

1. Extraordinary vessels, except the Ren and Du channels, are not visible in a healthy body that is in a state of balance. In other words, the regular meridians are balanced with Qi and smooth blood flow. If the body has an imbalance of hormonal or homeostatic metabolism, various abnormal symptoms or an accumulation on the eight extraordinary channels, will be present, depending on the different pathogens involved.
2. Extraordinary vessels are related to the balance of homeostasis and metabolism.
3. Extraordinary vessels manifest the state of the nervous, endocrine, and circulatory systems.

The eight extraordinary vessels and eight principles pattern identifications connect and provide an understanding of the body's homeostatic balancing system.

5

Six Body Types

PURPOSE OF DIFFERENTIATION

- Development of clear goals and plans of treatment
- Patient education for understanding of their state of conditions, treatments, and result
- Help to prevent next stage of disorder and maintain health

BACKGROUND

Typology is not appropriate for the treatment of patients, because each person has a different condition and is exposed to a different environment. However, the scope of practice with an acupuncture license supports a limited range of diagnostic tools and treatment methods. We need an integrated and open-minded approach to treatment. The six body type categories form the basis for selecting a treatment. These body types allow the practitioner to design a treatment and education plan for their patients.

The idea of six body types is based on the body's ability to adapt to homeostatic imbalance. During observation and treatment of patients concerned about sudden body changes, such as gaining weight, skin disorders, or the symptoms of bad postural pain, similar body structure patterns were found in similar symptoms and signs underlying a certain disorder, such as metabolic syndrome. It was noticed that internal organ disorders and external trauma affect the body structure and show the symptoms on superficial skin parts, which is explained as the traditional Chinese medicine (TCM) meridian function. It is further known that the meridian can transmit the treatment effect to internal organs. Therefore, if we change the body structure that has been adapted according to the dysfunction, the health state of the internal organ system and body function will change.

59

Six body types are based on these ideas.

- Weight gain is not the state of adding the mass of fat.
- Consider local fat deposits and local body obesity that may have internal problems.
- Superficial meridian and a wide range of meridians present the internal conditions.
- Aligned and balanced meridians can help to organize the body structure and function with behavior change.
- Although all meridians are important for six body types treatment, the muscle meridian, cutaneous meridian, and eight extraordinary vessel meridians are used for interpretation and treatment.

These six body types are differentiated based on TCM meridian aspects and determine the treatment plan and methods. With limited treatment tools and methods, some patterns have been developed in clinical practice.

TREAT BRANCHES AND ROOT

Chronic disorders or diseases need to have many hours of visits for treating the root cause, not the symptoms. However, we are able to deal with the symptoms, such as pain, in a short time. It is crucial that the practitioner determine the cause, as the signs and symptoms are merely the tip of the proverbial iceberg. The cause and effect are always bound together, even though there may be a chicken and egg situation. Understanding the causes may allow a chance to prevent secondary disorders. Once the cause is determined and the cycle of poor health is understood, the first step to restore health has been taken. It needs constant effort through medical care and changing the environment and an individual's behavior. Patients need to be patient.

When the symptoms are not considered serious, but the patient is not feeling well, we start to source solutions from alternative therapies or physical exercises, or nutritional supplements. There are certain types of patterns in the body that indicate the source of the problem. If we understand our body, then it will be easier to make the correct choices about our body and health.

CRITERIA OF THE SIX BODY TYPES

These criteria are neither a fixed condition nor a permanent symptom group; they can be changeable and manifested according to the degree of the problem. These different types help to solve the puzzle of defining the correct treatment. The six body types are

- Body structural (anatomical) groups—M1, M2, M3
- Body function (physiologic) groups—P, T, S

The first three body types are classified by looking (inspection) and palpating diagnostic methods and are based on an anatomical approach. The latter three types are differentiated by physiologic features (Figure 5.1).

Six Body Types • 61

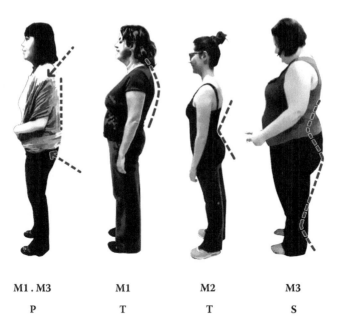

M1 . M3   M1   M2   M3
P   T   T   S

FIGURE 5.1
Body types.

Types M1, M2, and M3 are represented by the structural disorder related to upper, middle, and lower body parts. Types P, T, and S are the progressive sequential disorder, which means that type P can develop to become type T and then type S. They include body shape, movement, walking gait, range of motion, and objective pain when palpating the concerned spot. There are four major diagnostic procedures during each session of treatment, as well as during the first office visit. The four pillars of diagnosis are looking, listening, questioning, and palpating.

Since complementary and alternative therapies are major tools in this diagnostic and treatment design, both patients and practitioners should understand the level of health status. If severe signs and symptoms of an aggravating disorder are detected, it is important that the practitioner recommend the patient seek appropriate specialist treatment.

CHARACTERISTICS OF THE SIX BODY TYPES

- Mutual interconnection
- Shows at least one or more characteristics
- Treatment should follow the order of major types if multiple types are shown

Before beginning an explanation of the six body types, several characteristics must be introduced first. These characteristics are mutually interconnected and interrelated with each other. For example, if type M1 is diagnosed as the dominant and major issue, sometimes the treatment for body reshaping will start with type P, because the temporal or chronic issue from type M1 brings on the tension pain, and type P treatment will be a better choice for the pressure pain.

Since body system and functions have a remarkable ability to adapt, several types may present at the same time. If multiple types are presented, the treatment will follow the order of later occurring symptoms in the major type.

TYPE P (FIGURE 5.2)

Quick Tips

- You feel uncomfortable or lazy when you are calm and doing nothing.
- You feel bloated and have gained weight. You think that vigorous activities are the only solution; however, this is only effective if you are in your 20s.
- At night, a glass of wine, a favorite alcohol or snack, or making love right before bedtime can help to relieve stress and induce a good night's sleep.

- You have shoulder or neck pain when you wake up in the morning, especially if you partied and drank the previous evening or even two days ago.
- You are big on laughter. You frequently indulge in loud laughing even though the incident or conversation was not funny. Or you suddenly want to talk to someone and do not want to wait.
- You experience frequent feelings of heat in the chest or face.
- Your upper body is fat, rather than your extremities.
- Do you have a project or test that is due now?
- Do you think you need more sleep in the morning?
- You have chronic pain but do not bother with pain medication.
- You have frequently injured arms and legs.
- You keep saying how busy and tired you are but never slow down.
- You smoke.
- You really enjoy a back and shoulder massage.

Related Conditions

- Tension headache
- Dry mouth, dry eyes, and dry skin condition
- Pain in right side of shoulder and neck
- Ankle and wrist pain or tendonitis
- Shortness of breath or dizziness
- Palpitations in chest and back
- Cold hands and feet or static skin disorder
- Stress-induced autoimmune disorder
- Bloating and constipation
- Menstrual cramping
- Hernia or hemorrhoids
- Acne on face and body

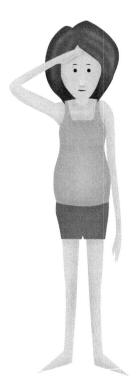

FIGURE 5.2
Type P.

- Sensitive to light, sound, and smell
- Anxiety, but not depression
- Hair loss
- Hypertension

Clinical Syndrome

Type P has four major patterns:

- Body trunk pressed (strong, tense, or congested) and extremities depressed (weak, flabby, or dry)
- Body trunk depressed (weak, flabby, or dried) and extremities pressed (strong, tensed, or accumulated)
- Skin tension—muscle weak
- Skin weak—muscle tension

Like our breathing rhythm, our body follows rhythmic motion and balance, such as contraction and relaxation of the heart muscle, inhalation and exhalation as in breathing, in-and-out exchange of body fluids and blood vessels, ingestion and excretion in the digestive system, activity and rest, and wakefulness and sleep. TCM explains this active motion as yin and yang.

Once you have a yang stage, then you need a yin stage of similar duration. The balancing beat goes yin yang yin yang yin yang yin yang, like chukka chukka choo choo, chukka chukka choo choo. The predictable patterns provide stability and a feeling of security. If the pattern is yin yang yin yang yang yang yang yang yang yin yang yang yang, you will feel a little unstable and irritated. Our body also wants to feel secure and safe from the external environment, which is explained by the circadian rhythm, day and night.

According to TCM theory, the blood flows to the extremities for activity during the day and back to the organs in the trunk area at night, provided the body is in a state of health.

This means that during the daytime, the sympathetic system is dominant, while the parasympathetic system is dominant at night. Most skeletal muscles are relaxed in the parasympathetic mode, except the diaphragm.

Sympathetic and parasympathetic nerves form the autonomic nervous system, and the body switches the appropriate system on automatically. Type P patterns indicate a broken automatic systemic pattern.

Body Trunk Pressed and Extremities Depressed

Most common weight concern cases in type P are due to lack of sleep. Patients state that they want to lose weight, but are too busy to exercise, too busy to bathe, and too busy to cook. Yet they need to talk to friends, search for something, and think something for something. They never pause their busy mind and actually feel too overwhelmed to act physically.

They used to be active and athletic; however, their now-sedentary lifestyle triggered the physical changes, such as a bloated feeling in the abdomen and chest, shoulder and neck pain, and headaches. The bloated feeling is often accompanied by palpitations in the chest and upper back and night sweats.

If this condition continues, the face swells and the neck and chest become unusually enlarged. A fasting diet and exercise are then selected as a means to lose weight. Initially, a diet is preferable to exercise. This body type usually presents with type M1 yin postural problems involving the breathing muscles.

Body Trunk Depressed and Extremities Pressed

The other pattern of weight concerned in type P is lack of freedom. This type of life rhythm pattern is sedentary due to mental stress, for example, yin yin yang yin yin yang yin yang yang yang yang yang. This type used to relax and claim that their lifestyle was not very active. However, sudden incidents in life, such as a promotion, a big project, parenting, and commitments, can affect emotional alertness.

In this case, physical characteristic change and swollen tension are observable in all extremities and the palms and soles are sweaty. The trunk area will be very tight, and neck pain is a common complaint. Fat deposits are usually concentrated around the armpit and inguinal area, but later the swollen fatty tissue deposits spread toward the arms and legs.

These people complain that their arms and legs are bigger in proportion to their bodies. They want to lose fat on the back of their arms and inner thigh area. Rarely, types M1 and M3 present with structure problems, but in most cases, the body posture is not involved.

The individuals in this group can return to prior good health once they are able to spend time relaxing and engage in gentle balancing therapies, such as massage therapy.

Skin Tension—Muscle Weak

When we use our muscles or maintain posture, we need a tensional power to maintain structure and motion. The internal tension is mostly contributed by blood flow. During exercise, the blood goes to skeletal muscles in the relaxed phase. Contracting and relaxing muscles send the blood to the heart. However, a static posture while sitting or standing leads to local body fluids becoming congested, which results in skin tension and muscle weakness. This is due to lack of physical activity.

These patients present with swollen lower legs, upper back and neck area, arm triceps, and abdominal area. This condition is not serious until the skin is damaged or tears, such as in the case of stretch marks. Whenever the body structure changes or gains weight, the skin and muscles are warned of the expected damage and problems. One of the symptoms is cold arms and legs, and patients are usually sensitive to cold or hot. If you discover abnormal superficial skin tension, the muscles below tend to be lengthened and weak. This condition will develop into type T or type S if it becomes chronic.

Skin Weak—Muscle Tension

This type is found in the pattern of people who are very active and exercise on a regular basis. Some people even smoke and drink while they maintain other healthy habits. The skin remains loose in the presence of weight loss and toned muscles. They are hyperactive and hyper in emotion, too. Irritable and agitated feelings are often present, and they dislike to be controlled. They have tension headaches, tendonitis, temporomandibular joint (TMJ) problems, and facial and muscle pain. This type is due to lack of peripheral blood circulation.

Instead of overall fat deposits, the problem areas, such as tendonitis, can be due to accumulated body fluids that are difficult for the skin to control. The outer shape has cellulite and is bumpy, while the skin is dark. If the body is wrinkled or there is a loosened skin area, you will discover that the muscles beneath are hard and contracted. Since the peripheral blood circulation is not good, the distal body parts are affected and peripheral neuropathy and circulation problems present, such as cold hands and feet. This group of people experience chronic pain or trauma, so treating the chronic pathogenic factor needs to be carried out prior to weight loss treatment.

Understanding the Mechanism

Type P is defined as a chronic physical or mental stress state (Figure 5.3).

Stress responses and reactions vary between individuals. Any stressful situation, environmentally, physically, or emotionally, produces an acute disturbance in the body and an immediate reaction that places the autonomic nervous system in a flight or fight situation and the sympathetic nerves dominate. While it appears that the body is aware of a life-threatening and emergency situation, the body also reacts to small distresses, such as meeting a new person, making a presentation or a public speech, embarrassment, excitement, driving in heavy traffic, and exercise. Once alarmed, sympathetic responses occur very quickly as an entire body reaction, but return to normal or a relaxed mode once the situation is resolved. If the stressor is lifelong or is a repetitive activity, it maintains the body in chronic sympathetic mode.

A stress situation demonstrates that the body is made up of a great team of players.

Skeletal Muscles

The activation of sympathetic nerves results in initial stage vasoconstriction in the skeletal muscles. However, when doing exercise, in contrast, increasing the metabolic activity of muscle fibers induces vasodilation, because the contracting muscles produce their own insulin-like effect, causing the rapid uptake of glucose from the blood.

If you are doing exercise, your skeletal muscle brings the glucose from your blood vessels. As we know, physical exercise is recommended for those suffering from diabetes for this reason.

Even though you are in mental stress, the blood flow in skeletal muscles changes rapidly. They are ready to run or fight. If you sit all through a stressful day, and think that by going to bed you will finally relax, you are wrong. Your muscles' business is not done yet. The sleep will not be smooth. Rather, take a walk for a while or take a warm bath with Epsom salts to help your stressed muscles.

Simply stated, once you are in a state of stress, you need to use your skeletal muscles, which are already contracted and want to use the blood sugar. If you have a stress situation, move around, clean the house, or go for a walk, instead of trying to calm down. That is the best way of preventing weight gain.

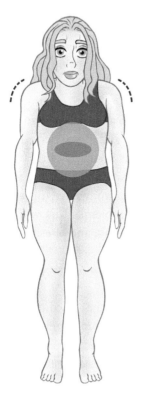

FIGURE 5.3
Type P mechanism.

Blood Vessels in Skin and Skeletal Muscle

Once the body has been stressed physically (including exercise) and mentally, the blood vessels dilate in the cardiac and skeletal muscles, but not in the gut system and skin, which are closer to the peripheral blood vessels in terms of their function. During stress on the body, they shunt blood away from the skin and extremities so that it can be used in parts more vital to survival. Then you see who the teammates are: heart and skeletal muscle versus gut and skin.

Even though we exercise for health, we sometimes focus too much on cardio and muscle strengthening, which results in the gut and skin being neglected. While muscle tone and blood circulation are important, the gut and skin are important for immune responses and nutrition.

In TCM, the skin is a reflection of the digestive system, so skin conditions are indicative of digestive system conditions. Before treating the skin disorder, pay attention to treating the gut system. Herbal bath therapy is recommended for helping the venous circulation, which affects the digestion.

Exercise helps to build muscle and maintain a look of health—while you are still young. However, some day, your skin will suddenly look old, even though you are still maintaining healthy muscles. Because your body was continually stressed in the sympathetic mode, your gut and skin were not nourished. If you want healthy skin and muscle tone, you need to plan a balanced lifestyle.

Breathing and Circulation = Air and Food

During an emergency, the airway, breathing, and circulation are the three basic principles for saving life. In daily life, they are also important for the maintenance and performance of the body. In Chapter 4, circulation and respiratory homeostatic functions were mentioned in detail. Circulation and breathing actions take place at the same time during homeostatic regulation. And the most important function of circulation is the distribution of nutrition to cells and the cellular respiratory action.

When you are hungry or eat too little, your body will bend forward, allowing breathing to strike a balance between thoracic and abdominal cavity pressure. If you eat too much and feel bloated, you will push out your abdomen and stretch the chest backward for a comfortable posture to breath. Our body automatically controls tension adjustment between the two cavities.

However, if one of them has been dominant and in a chronic phase, such as holding your breath from stress, or craving for overeating due to stress, the body shows the current conditions as upper chest tightness or big belly tension shape posture. To facilitate breathing and circulation, all the torso muscles remain neutral and loose, free to contract and relax because most torso muscles are involved with breathing and digestion. If you make your torso muscles too tight, you may have digestive issues or breathing problems. This will lead to congestion, swelling, and obesity.

Pain

Tension headache is common in type P patients. Symptoms include a tight feeling or a pulling and pushing pulsation on or around the head like a band. Once the headache starts, agitation and shortness of breathing are experienced. Lying down alleviates the pain.

Tension headaches sometimes come with shoulder pain and neck pain on one side, especially the right side. When you have a tension headache or right-side shoulder and neck pain, palpate the right side of your body. If you compare the left and right sides, you will notice that one side is more tense and shortened.

This type of pain is frequently found in sympathetic-induced constriction, and may arise during sudden emotional disturbance, such as anger or overeating, while drinking alcohol, in the presence of sleep disorders, and in cold weather.

Once you have a tension-related pain, the priority is "deflating your inner tension balloon."

Step 1: Open your mouth.
Step 2: Only focus on exhaling (breath out–breath in = 5:1).
Step 3: Loosen your all joints.
Step 4: Wriggle your fingertips and toes.
Step 5: Drink warm water or tea.

You will feel much better after these five steps, especially if you burp or release gas.

Postural Characteristics

Type P posture is similar to type M1, which is presented as bent forward upper chest, with arms and face in a boxer's position. The difference is the chin position and neck wrinkles. Type M1 tends to be chin up with one prominent wrinkle on the back of the neck, whereas type P shows as chin down and two or more wrinkles on the neck. Their facial expression is quite simple: serious expression and artificial smile, artificial smile and serious expression, with crying when needed.

If types P and M2 are combined, skin tension is prominent. If the condition is combined with type M3, the spinal curve is reduced and a long torso shape is presented.

Possible Associated Disorders

- Tension headache
- Hyperthyroidism
- Hypertension
- Diabetes mellitus
- Posttraumatic stress disorder (PTSD)

Treatment

Body trunk pressed and extremities depressed
- Open chest and pull down on abdominal tension.
- Acupuncture treatment required on pectoralis major and minor and rotator cuff muscles.
- Gastrointestinal resuscitation (GIR) direction on lower section and heat on upper middle section on abdomen.

Body trunk depressed and extremities pressed
- Loosen extremity joints and muscle.
- Acupuncture treatment required on distal points of extremities (popular points are Lv3 and Li4: between the first and second metatarsal and metacarpal areas).
- Moxa oil gua sha distal to medial scraping.

Skin tension—muscle weak
- Hyperthermal therapy.
- Find the depressed area and apply muscle meridian needling on the lines or area.

Skin weak—muscle tension
- Skin stimulation therapy, such as moxa oil scraping on the skin until it turns red.

- Find the tension spot between the muscle and tendon.
- Standing on tread needling technique on tension line.

Simple Home Therapy and Caution

There are three different reactions and secretions from our body during intense stress. For example, public speaking is a form of stress and may induce anxiety and fear. At that moment, serum epinephrine activates from the adrenal gland. Epinephrine is the "flight" level of sympathetic neurotransmitter and hormone that may induce loss of control in a stress situation.

However, when you do physical exercise, the rise of the serum level of norepinephrine leads to a controllable stress situation, or "fight."

Another stress hormone, cortisol, is engaged in chronic stage stress and makes you feel defeated and hopeless. That is why chronic pain syndrome accompanies the psychological issue.

Type P patients are usually very active and busy. They are afraid of relaxing and calming even though they want to be relaxed. Since sympathetic and parasympathetic nervous systems are autonomic, they are not aware of autonomic responses, nor do they change with willpower.

However, we can try to change the environment with some mechanism input to emotions and visceral sensory information, such as smell, taste, temperature, and osmolality of blood, since the hypothalamus is the major controller. For this reason, when treating type P, gastrointestinal resuscitation and hyperthermal therapy are applied during the first few sessions and then facial muscle and neck treatments follow.

Even though the sympathetic flight or fight mode responds with one push of the button, the parasympathetic mode "rest and digest" has many buttons to be pushed before a response occurs. A relaxed mode may be induced by listening to familiar music, smelling a pleasant fragrance, engaging in warm cuddles, having craniosacral therapy or mild cupping on the back, getting a gentle massage, taking a warm bath, or singing a song.

Case Study

The case study involves a 48-year-old female whose main complaint was tension headache.

Brief History

The patient visited my clinic four years ago. When I first saw her, she appeared very tired and desperate. For almost seven years, she had been suffering from severe idiopathic headaches. An MRI revealed no abnormalities. She took strong pain medication whenever she had a headache. Once the headache flared up, she reported that it continued for several hours to several days.

She operated a business during the afternoon and evening. During business hours, she wore high heels and dressed up. Her bedtime was around 2:00–3:00 a.m. and she woke up around 10:00 a.m. Her sleep quality was good unless the headache flared up. She does not have any children. She drank alcohol frequently.

Except for the headaches, she did not have other issues and concerns regarding health, but she did not like abdominal fat and underwent a liposuction procedure twice several years previously. She said that her abdominal area was flat immediately after surgery, but the side of the body started becoming bigger than before. Recently, she felt very fat and was depressed as a result.

She injured her left arm during childhood, a mild tear in the ligaments in the shoulder area. That was the only issue of concern.

Observations

The first impression was that of dry skin and hair, and ballooning body shape with tension. She appeared overweight, but her skin, hair, and complexion were very dry. She constantly frowned, displaying wrinkles between the eyebrows. When I asked the location of the headache, she indicated almost her entire head. Her head, face, and even neck looked swollen, but it did not look like water retention, nor did her head feel wet. Her scalp felt abnormal when I palpated her head, as though a soft blanket covered her head.

She had several small scars from liposuction surgery on the side of her abdomen. Her rib cage was wide open; the angle of the xyphoid was more than 120°. Her chest was very swollen, and it was difficult to distinguish the rib bones and clavicles. Abdominal tension made her jump whenever I touched with a light pressure. The abdominal area was very flat but widely opened and stretched. When she lay down, her abdomen was depressed, but in the standing posture, her abdomen protruded forward.

Her arms and legs were lean and weak. Her upper chest and facial neck were large and swollen, whereas the extremities were thin and weak. She had two wrinkles on the back of her neck, and the area between the wrinkles was swollen. Her skin was dry, but without further indication of disorder. Her legs were straight and the body structures were fine.

Assessments and Plan

This case can be classified as types P and M1. Since she had an injured arm, her habit of carrying and lifting items had changed since her childhood. She had used her chest, neck, and even TMJ when she carried heavy items to compensate for the power distribution.

As she did not have much time for physical activities and exercise, her extremities and skeletal muscles were weak and lean. As a result, most tension gathered in the trunk area, especially the chest. Her physical stress from standing and working all day and lack of sleep led to chronic fatigue and digestive problems. That led to abdominal fat congestion due to poor breathing and circulation.

After the liposuction, her chronic pain response to touch and pressure resulted in her body adopting a posture to avoid the pain. The raised shoulder and shallow breathing occurred because of the abdominal tension. Poor breathing and circulation can cause a swollen body, even in the upper chest and head.

Abdominal muscle tightness limited diaphragm movement, so overall, her body was rigid and tight. Alcohol affected her blood vessels and inflamed her body. Chronic body fluid congestion in her upper chest and neck area also prevented the restoration of muscle and tendon function.

Although headache is her main complaint, her body indicated that she needed to be treated for other causative factors.

The initial treatment was for type M1: breathing muscle and neck muscle area were loosened to facilitate circulation and help breathing. Since her abdominal area was sensitive and painful on the surface, her back and side were treated with hyperthermal methods instead of GIR to relax her body.

After several sessions, her abdominal area remained tight but her headache was relieved. The key to relieving the headache was releasing neck muscle and congested fat tissue on the back of neck area. The breathing muscles and armpit congestion were treated.

Type P patient home care is important for maintaining the treatment results. She was recommended a half-body bath and a small-portion diet. Several months later, her neck and facial swelling had subsided, the symptoms of headache were gone, and her waistline and weight had been reduced. Her trousers size decreased from size 8 to 2. She has been treated for her condition for about three years, once a week.

TYPE T (FIGURE 5.4)

Quick Tips

- You are sensitive to changes in weather or dislike hot or cold sensations. Someone opens the window and you immediately are cold and angry with the person who opened it. You wear several items of clothing, socks, and muffler.
- Do you recently feel lonely or depressed despite the fact that you have family, friends, and pets? You feel alone in a crowd.
- Are you afraid of being among many people at a gathering or in society? You worry about catching a cold, especially during the common cold or viral season. You really do not like to see your coworkers sick because you do not want to become sick from a contagious disease.
- Are you interested in new diets because whatever you eat makes you uncomfortable? You think that your digestion issues are from food selections.
- Someone asks a favor of you, but you think, "I can't be bothered."
- You do not care for your appearance, such as your waistline, skin, or clothing; you just want to be healthy because you have been suffering from minor ailments.
- You have allergy symptoms: itching eyes, runny nose, heartburn-like sore throat, and skin allergy from weather change.
- Whenever you feel fatigue and tired, your skin problem irritates you more.

Related Conditions

- Cold sensitivity
- Fatigue and depression
- Food intolerance
- Constipation or loose stool
- Irritated skin condition
- Severe allergy symptoms (not specific with allergen)

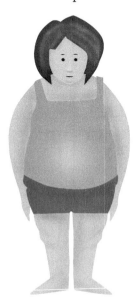

FIGURE 5.4
Type T.

- Distal joint pain and weakness (fingers, wrists, toes, ankles)
- Facial swelling and arm skin condition (chicken skin: keratosis pilaris)
- Feeling heavy and weight gain
- Frequent infection and inflammation
- Taking several nutritional supplements or herbs
- Recent blood test that is slightly low or high in the normal range

Clinical Syndrome

The type T group tends to visit health practitioners because of their health and appearance changes, whereas the type P group is more self-contained to figure out their health concerns, such as exercise, diet, meditation, nutritional supplements, and visiting a spa. If type P is manifested in the imbalance of body rhythm, type T is the broken cycle reaction in the body system, especially the metabolic pathway (Figure 5.5). Type T is a more chronic stage than type P is, and is mostly manifested in autonomic nervous system imbalance. If the symptom is not resolved, the symptoms and signs will begin to diversify.

The metabolic homeostasis has been disturbed due to autonomic nervous system imbalance. For maintaining metabolic homeostasis, the nervous, endocrine, and vascular systems are all integrated. Metabolism requires chemical balance, oxygen level balance, correct temperature for enzymes, and proper removal of waste products.

Type T patients visit for treatment of the digestive system, skin eczema, and allergic reactions, especially temperature-triggered allergic symptoms. Some people are diagnosed by medical doctors as having fibromyalgia chronic pain syndrome or functional gastrointestinal disorder.

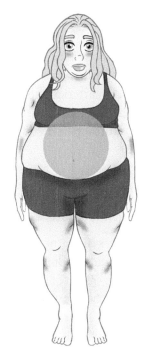

FIGURE 5.5
Type T mechanism.

Type T is defined by the following patterns:

- Lymphatic body fluid congestion involving inflammation with the group of symptoms
- Skeletal muscle weakness from eccentric contraction; cannot push to return venous and lymphatic system
- Weakness of thoracic inspiration due to chronic physical stress that fails to help lymphatic function

Most lymph flow in the body depends on the contracting skeletal muscles and breathing movements, especially the inspiration resulting from diaphragm descent. Lymph flow is very slow and one directional to the central venous system through the thoracic duct. This movement is against gravity. Overall, the average volume of lymph that enters the venous system is about three liters.

Vigorous activity, exercise, and heavy load breathing can help to move lymph flow. But if a physical activity is not allowed, then we need to find other pressure-generating aids. It can be an arterial pulsation, changing posture, or passive compression, such as acupressure, massage, and gua sha.

Understanding the Mechanism

Immune System Lymph

The lymphatic system not only prevents harmful body fluid buildup in our body, but also prevents the spread of disease. Most systems of the body benefit from the lymphatic system with the balancing of fluids and immune functions. The lymph defense system fights against microorganism and disease by filtering them through the lymph nodes and destroying them with lymphocytes that migrate from blood vessels to lymph vessels. The defense system is widespread in the body, protecting major organs from external pathogens located in the four extremities and neck and internal organ systems such as the lungs and intestines.

For this reason, we can notice the localized or whole-body swelling or water accumulation on the area, which can be a minor inflammation or severe trauma, like a burn. Even hormone changes can affect the lymph system, such as menstrual swelling, because with every small change in the body, normal homeostatic function tries to adapt to the new circumstance, which leads to activation of the homeostatic control system and negative feedback.

Transportation of Nutrient: Lymph System

During digestion, the small particles of food broken down from digestive hormones are absorbed in mostly the small intestine and transported to the bloodstream. Larger particles, such as fat, are transported by the lacteal gland, which is the lymph vessel, from the abdominal wall to the larger lymph system, cisterna chyli.

The lymph sac, cisterna chyli, is affected by diaphragm pressure, which means that the transport of the fat nutrients is affected by diaphragmatic breathing. When you are in a stressful sedentary lifestyle or after having a big meal, you may feel the palpitation on the upper abdominal area while lying down. The cisterna chyli is located in the lower back near the aorta.

In clinical experience, the individual suffering allergies and lymph drainage blocking conditions presents with midback bending posture and spinal muscle tightness (T11–L2).

In TCM, the spleen's main function is within the nutritional transportation system. If spleen Qi is weak, initially, lack of appetite, abdominal distension after eating, fatigue, loose stool, and shallow complexion are shown as symptoms. If it progresses to the chronic stage, dampness occurs, which leads to nausea, feeling stuffiness in the chest, and heaviness in the extremities. Treatments are specifically related to each condition. It can also be developed as a spleen yang deficiency. The spleen yang deficiency symptoms are added cold feeling and dampness in the body (edema), including all spleen Qi deficiency symptoms.

The epigastric area is packed with organs, large blood vessels, and important glands. In addition, the nutrients' lymphatic fluids are waiting for the diaphragmatic action. If it is not working properly, epigastric congestion may occur, and can restrict breathing muscle movement. Once the breathing and circulation system is altered, then the thermoregulatory mechanism starts to change.

Unlike other yang deficiencies, spleen yang deficiency directly affects widespread edema due to the involvement of the respiratory and circulatory system.

Lymph Fluid Accumulation

Another important role of the lymphatic system is to transport proteins from the interstitial space within a tissue or organ. If the transport capacity of the lymphatic system is reduced, proteins and other substances accumulate in the interstitium (an interstitial space within a tissue or organ). Especially, accumulated proteins attract water, which creates high-protein swelling in the subcutaneous tissues, called lymphedema.

Lymphedema is a slow-onset condition occurring when body systems recover from accidents, trauma, chronic disorder, or progressive disease characterized by an asymmetrical, inflammatory swelling traveling distal to proximal. Any body part may be affected, including limbs, trunk, head and neck, and even the genitals.

This condition involves capillary blood vessels and lymphatic vessels. Drainage is one of the lymph system's roles. While collecting the extracellular water (including waste products, dead cells, and bacteria), lymph vessels tend to be accompanied with veins, except in the abdominal cavity. The lymph and venous system depend on skeletal muscle movement because they do not have their own pump to reach the upper cervical area. Thus, healthy muscle tone, adequate movement during the day, full range of diaphragmatic breathing, and peripheral blood circulation are important to prevent accumulation of lymph fluid in the body. Prevention for the accumulation of body fluids includes

- Healthy muscles (neutral state, ability to relax and contract)
- Active body work, movement, action, and exercise
- Good quality of breathing and blood circulation
- A good source of nutrition and a healthy digestive system
- For a healthy digestive system, adequate rest and sleep time

Venous Insufficiency

Skeletal muscle movement pump action is an important factor for venous return, as well as lymphatic fluid movement. Venous return occurs with skeletal muscle pump in the extremities and respiratory activity in the abdominal thoracic area. If it is not working properly, venous insufficiency begins in the legs, which are swollen, skin is darkened (hyperpigmentation), skin thickening occurs (lipodermatosclerosis), or an ulcer forms near the ankle.

Individuals from the type T group present with swollen legs and vein problems, such as spider veins and varicose veins, in the initial stages. If this condition is not resolved, the muscle will change to a string-like shape and painful tension will build up in the leg and ankle area. This leads the walking-gait limitation of the feet.

Gaining Weight

You have been busy, with not much time to take care of yourself. Long-term disturbances made your immune system weak and gave you a minor disorder. Hovering between well-being and disease, you can continue your stressful daily life, but you feel tired and overwhelmed. This is the point where we are blocked from seeing our own appearance. We are too busy to see the mirror, too busy to check the waist, and too busy to treat a headache. Gaining weight is not because of your lazy lifestyle or eating too much. You did not have a chance to take care of your inner or outer broken cycle and rhythm.

Pain

Individuals in type T do not complain of pain during the initial stage. The more concerning issues are fatigue, allergy reaction, skin problems, and digestive issues. While they visit my clinic and have treatment for those issues, the pain symptoms occur from an unexpected area or whole-body pain. This happens frequently in acupuncture clinics. After treatment, patients have body pain and feel weak and tired. Since type T usually progresses to type P, due to broken biorhythm, the body has been holding the tension and stress chronically and cannot resolve it or move to the relaxed stage by themselves.

This happens during the weekend after intense and stressful work, or vacation sickness after a long-term project is completed. The symptoms are usually shown as cold, allergy, or whole-body ache. Type T patients need to be instructed and informed about what symptoms to expect after treatments. If the body has been stressed for a long time, the hyperstage becomes normal for the body. So, even though the body does go into a relaxed stage, the person feels ill or depressed in his or her hyperadapted body. This body pain is not too severe in its first occurrence, but later it possibly develops to

chronic fatigue syndrome (CFS) or fibromyalgia if accompanied with hormone changes or body fluid loss in certain conditions.

CFS is a disorder that causes you to become so fatigued (tired) you cannot perform normal daily tasks. This is called chronic fatigue. The main symptom of CFS is chronic fatigue that lasts more than six months. Physical or mental activities often make the symptoms worse, and rest usually does not improve the symptoms.

People who have CFS may experience the following symptoms:

- Fatigue
- Headaches
- Sore throat
- Tender or painful areas in the neck or armpits due to swollen lymph nodes (or lymph glands)
- Muscle soreness
- Pain that moves from joint to joint without swelling or redness
- Loss of memory or concentration
- Trouble sleeping
- Extreme tiredness after exercising that lasts more than 24 hours

These and other symptoms often will not go away or keep coming back for six months or more.

CFS may occur after an illness (such as a cold), or it can start during or shortly after a period of high stress. It can also come on slowly without any clear starting point or any obvious cause. In some cases, CFS can last for years.

In TCM, this stage arises from spleen Qi deficiency and damp accumulation, which leads to the dense formed condition of phlegm with heat-generating form, the continued chronic stress. In other words, damp heat easily dries up body fluids and condenses it as phlegm. There are two different phlegm categories, substantial and insubstantial phlegm. Substantial phlegm is visible, such as when coughing or vomiting. Insubstantial phlegm is often the consequence of internal disruption of the body's fluid metabolism.

Once phlegm has occurred in the body, the pathogens will be unpredictable and will involve various symptoms, so it is known as a notorious pathogen to treat and diagnose because it results from the disturbance of homeostatic balance and affects metabolic homeostasis.

Postural Characteristics

The first impression of type T is a "square" body shape, and the extremities are weak and thin, whether the person is lean or looks overweight. This is because his or her lymph body fluids are congested and the lymphatic drainage system is affected. The upper back, armpits, lower abdomen to thigh, and side of the body are the major congestion areas. He or she may have a forward stoop, but this is not related to spinal deformity such as kyphosis, but looks as though the entire body leans forward, including neck and head.

Possible Associated Disorders

- Chronic fatigue syndrome
- Fibromyalgia
- Multiple chemical sensitivities
- Chronic mononucleosis
- Orthostatic intolerance
- Irritable bowel syndrome
- Interstitial cystitis
- TMJ pain
- Chronic pelvic pain

Treatment

Type T patients are treated with "press and depress" methods in my clinic. They include hydrostatic pressure, negative pressure, releasing muscle tension, tightening of the skin, and encouraging emotion from the depression.

The stage of type T is the next level of type P which is dominated from stress stage. Unresolved tension is due to chronic inflammation or local congestion, which is shown as swollen or depressed surfaces. Sometimes patients think that it is "fat" on their back, thighs, or arms. However, the area has a tight muscle or scar tissue underneath and the gap between the skin and muscle is thicker than in other parts of the body. That is the point of muscle meridian needling. Type T is influenced on foot yang muscle tendon meridians.

In understanding the structure, type M2 has been introduced as inner tension pushed out to exterior surfaces and the body outer shell being adapted as the transformation of the spine and skin area. Type T is the opposite action. The outer surface's congestion and tension buildup tend to push inward and restrict the normal movement inside, especially the digestive and respiratory systems.

For example, the stretch mark is usually on the surface area from the tension of internal change, such as pregnancy or local swelling. After resolving the internal congestion or delivery, the stretch mark areas remain as the depressed extra skin surface initially, and then later, they gradually build up as thick tight tissue, which can restrict the inner functional movement, such as breathing. Therefore, the chronic stage of type T treatment is similar to that of type M2.

The digestive and respiratory systems are the core of the press and depress system.

Two major parts are treated at the same time. Type T symptoms and signs are presented as various and hard to distinguish at one glance. However, we cannot miss the important point for this syndrome from chronic stress, which can affect the digestive system and the circulatory breathing system.

The core treatment, restoring the digestive system, will be emphasized in type T. So, in each treatment session, facial and neck treatment or GIR treatment for restoring the digestive system is followed by muscle meridian treatment.

Type T treatment is not simple with a quick response. It takes several months to years, depending on the symptoms and signs.

Simple Home Care and Cautions

Type T is involved with many aspects of metabolic homeostatic function, and one or two factors are not working well. The important thing is that it took a long time for this stage to develop from a state of imbalance to where your body had adapted to its new environment. Therefore, it is unrealistic to expect quick results and big changes right away. However, if you do not give up, then your comfortable, healthy state will be restored. Keep this in mind as your long-term goal for your health.

Before your body adapts to its broken cyclic balance, you need to regulate it with habit change.

At first, the stressor is removed. If it is impossible to avoid it, you need to regulate your habit with other things instead.

For type T, nighttime is crucial for recovery of the basic metabolic system. Spend more time on yourself, at least 30 minutes every day. Fix your bedtime around 11:00 p.m. and before bedtime, you need to spend one hour of private time for you. Soak your feet in warm water, pamper your face and neck for a while, or take a warm half-body bath for 20 minutes until you have forehead sweat.

It may be not easy to have a good sleep every time; sometimes you will wake up at 2:00 a.m. or 3:00 a.m. It is fine, and do not worry about that since you will sleep well the next day. Do not take note of what time you wake up or how long you slept; you just need to focus on your fixed bedtime.

Breakfast is vital and your first meal should be solid food. You need to use your masseter muscle for mastication. Drinking only coffee, milk, or juice is not considered breakfast. Especially, if you feel muzzy in your head, struggle to concentrate, or have brain fog, you need to eat warm solid food at breakfast time. If you have been skipping breakfast and have no appetite in the morning, instead skip dinner or eat earlier in the evening from now on. The first several days will be challenging, but your body will adapt sooner than you expect. When it comes to meal portions, instead of a "bullying diet," reduce your portion sizes. Instead of using a dinner plate, switch to a dessert plate for all your meals.

For type T, exercise is not recommended until a few symptoms are relieved. Light walking or stretching can be enough physical exercise.

Case Study

The case study involves a 44-year-old female whose main complaints are allergies, runny nose, sneezing, body pain, and facial acne.

Brief History

She visited my clinic for reducing allergy symptoms that were present for about seven months and had worsened recently. She reported trying almost everything to relieve the symptoms. An allergy test did not indicate any specific allergen, but she had taken several injections and medications whenever allergies flared up.

Recently, she had other symptoms when waking up. It was difficult to do daily chores due to the heavy feeling of back pain and fatigue. A low energy level and body aches made her depressed.

She was very busy, worked for a company, and did volunteer social work during the weekend. She was very social and active. She had no history of surgery.

Her digestion was not good, but she did not care much about the digestion problems because other issues affected her health. Otherwise, she did not focus excessively on the issues.

Observations

Her complexion was dark, and acne was present on her forehead and the side of her cheeks. Her posture stooped forward from the midback. This was an extraordinary case. There was no flexibility. Her body shape was square, as though widely opened side by side, and it looked as though two people pulled her arms from each side.

Her skin looked dry and thick. When I palpated her back, it was difficult to reach the scapular and spinal bone, even though she was not obese or swollen. The skin and muscles were very tight and rigid. There was some local skin discoloration on the mid–upper back area. The rear side of her neck had two deep wrinkles.

Her hamstrings and gastrocnemius were weak and tender. Abdominal tension was connected with chest tightness. The chest skin had bumps like chicken skin, and the armpit area had darkened spots.

Her face had active acne on the forehead and cheeks and some old scars and dark spots. Overall, her face was swollen.

She was diagnosed in groups type T and type M2. Before developing as type T, she had been stressed and tensed on her trunk.

Since her legs and arms are aligned and back-of-neck wrinkles gave the two lines for the tension clue, her tension is assumed in her trunk area. Sometimes it is very difficult to find the origin of tension, especially when the patient does not want to discuss medical history or life pattern.

Her condition started in her 20s in college, in the coldest area in the United States. She was raised in tropical weather and moved to the northern East Coast area. Several times, she had severe cold and allergy symptoms, but they were not long lasting. She then moved to the West Coast and worked there. She felt tired, but she pushed forward toward her goal and belief. For about 20 years, she had barely been on vacation or taken time off for herself.

Although type T patients have various symptoms and signs, it is priority to find the origin of the most stressed tension spot. Her tension area was the epigastric area. From the epigastric area to the spine and rib cage, a deformed shape of body structure was present, which entailed a forward-protruding rib cage and back-side bandlike tissue accumulation. Since her main complaint was allergy, I tried to treat the symptoms as well as the tension treatment. I have been treating her for several years, and during this period, most of her major symptoms have disappeared. She visits on a regular basis for maintaining her body condition.

TYPE S (FIGURE 5.6)

Quick Tips

- Are you taking medications for blood pressure, diabetes, birth control, or hormonal therapy?
- Have you been overweight for a long time, or did you gradually change your size within five years?
- Have you been struggling to lose weight for at least five years? Are diet and exercise not working for losing weight? Do they sometimes make it worse?
- Before the change in body shape, were there severe digestive issues, chronic cold symptoms with immune deficiency, and long-term antibiotic use?
- Does fat deposit in specific areas, such as the shoulder and abdomen, but the condition is not bothersome to daily life? Do you sometimes have distending pain in your lower back and knee?
- Have you ever had major surgeries in your trunk area or lower abdomen?
- Do you take sleeping pills or antidepressant medication or herbs?
- Have you ever been diagnosed with a heart problem, kidney problem, or stroke?
- Has any trauma or accident occurred that needed a long recovery time?

Related Conditions

- Depression, anger, frustration, negative feeling
- Seems that exercise and diet do not help to lose weight and change lifestyle
- Feeling very tired, hard to control emotional outbursts
- Taking multivitamins and nutritional supplements due to fatigue, dizziness, pain, and sleep disorder
- Women: Hormone imbalance, infertility, irregular menstruation
- Lipedema: Hip, thigh, legs and arms, lower abdomen
- Arthritic pain on wrist and ankle: Possible start of rheumatoid arthritis symptoms on finger or toe
- Lower back pain from sitting; painful and swollen wrists and ankles when walking and using arms
- Postpartum depression and weight gain in the past
- Postsurgery and old scar tissue on trunk area

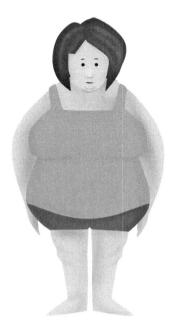

FIGURE 5.6
Type S.

- Metabolic syndrome
- Hypothalamic disorder
- Thyroid disorder and taking thyroid medication
- Drink alcohol frequently and shoulder pain next day

Clinical Syndrome

As the imbalance in metabolic homeostasis progresses, type P is related to autonomic nervous system rhythm, and it is represented as excess (hyper) and deficiency (hypo) and rest–digest and flight–fight. Type T is related with the metabolic homeostasis imbalance stage that is not stable and changes rapidly. It affects the body's immune system and shows as inflammatory responses and body fluid congestion. It is represented as hot (inflammation or fast acting) and cold (body fluid congestion, slow acting, or blocking). Regarding the type M group, types P, T, and S are distinguished as exterior conditions for type M, which is mostly considered to be related to posture, muscle, and skin parts. Moreover, types P, T, and S are explained by internal body condition.

Type S is the state in which the body has already adapted to the chronic imbalance condition.

This group of patients visits the clinic for weight loss rather than other issues. Unlike type T, type S patients start to talk about the other issues after several sessions. Both male and female patients have digestive issues and reproductive system issues.

Type S can be developed from types P and T, but if patients take medications, have experienced traumatic incidents, or have a genetic hormonal disorder, they show similar symptoms and signs.

Since types M1, M2, and M3 can be diagnosed at the same time as type S, and type P and type T are included in some patterns and ruled out in others, when taking the medical history and palpating, it is difficult to decide or diagnose the etiology in type S in the initial assessment. For this reason, I separate the subpatterns in clinical treatment assessment.

There are four different patterns in type S, which are differentiated by the etiology in symptomatic appearances. The name is from the eighth extraordinary meridian (vessel, Mai), which is the guideline and map of treatment.

1. Chong and yin Wei type (heart and digestive system)
2. Dai and yang Wei type (liver and immune system)
3. Ren and yin Qiao type (lung and circulatory system)
4. Du and yang Qiao type (kidney and nervous system)

Chong and Yin Wei Type (Heart and Digestive System) (Figure 5.7)

Characteristics

- Thoracic rib cage is wider and larger looking
- Weak and lean extremities
- Abdominal area tight
- Chest, neck, and face swollen

This condition is usually related to internal scar tissue blocking the blood vessel, or a structural problem that hinders blood circulation. Some cases have chronic digestive

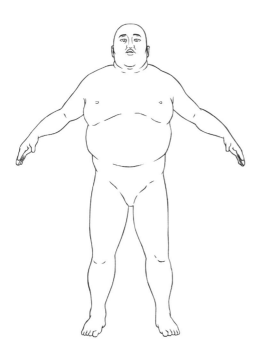

FIGURE 5.7
Chong and yin Wei type.

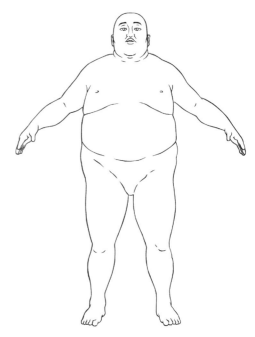

FIGURE 5.8
Dai and yang Wei type.

system issues and subsequent malnutrition. Type P and Type M1 yin are involved in this condition.

Dai and Yang Wei Type (Liver and Immune System) (Figure 5.8)

Characteristics

- Pear-shaped body
- Love handles
- Square shape of body appearance if leg muscles are misaligned
- Lower abdomen and hip area fat deposits

This condition is related to types T and M2. It is in the chronic stage, and body structure changed after childbirth or because of a liver disorder or visceral fat deposit condition. This appearance is shown as a lower back, side, and abdominal connection in a tube shape. The skin is usually stretched and irregular skin fat is present.

Ren and Yin Qiao Type (Lung and Circulatory System) (Figure 5.9)

Characteristics

- Abdominal tension and upper abdomen fat deposits
- Apple-shaped body
- X shape of legs
- Flat feet
- Shortness of breath

This type is related to types M2 and P. These types present with gynecological problems due to pelvic tilt, metabolic syndrome such as diabetes mellitus, and hypertension.

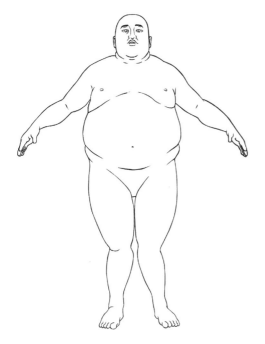

FIGURE 5.9
Ren and yin Qiao type.

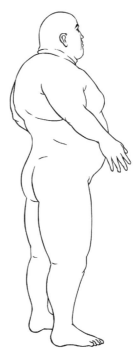

FIGURE 5.10
Du and yang Qiao type.

Du and Yang Qiao Type (Kidney and Nervous System) (Figure 5.10)

Characteristics

- Round shoulders and upper back fat deposits
- Smaller hips than upper back
- Lower abdominal fat but not prominent
- O shape of legs (bow legs)
- Hyperplantar flexion
- Short neck

Types M3 and P are related to this condition and result from nervous system and nerve balance disorder. Patients suffer from multiple disorders and take several medications and nutritional supplements for homeostatic dysfunction. During the initial visit, it is difficult to determine their type and how to approach treatment of their symptoms.

Male patients who are in type S show fat distribution on the lower abdomen and breast area. It is usually accompanied by childhood obesity. They have tried to lose weight with diet plans and exercise but cannot reduce the fat bulges. Female patients in type S are easily affected by emotional and physical distress from sudden environmental changes, such as gynecological surgery and the experience of a life-threatening ailment. An extremely stressful situation can be the trigger to the start of type S.

There are interesting patterns in type S, and in the midst of all the different triggers, the common symptom is digestive problems in early life or severe damage in the digestive system.

They avoid certain types of food, and during childhood, experienced food induced allergic reactions. Sometimes sleep disorders and hormonal imbalances are present.

Some patients have strong, chronic inflammatory symptoms.

Understanding the Mechanism

When a change occurs in an environment, an adjustment must be made in the body system. The receptors sense the changes in the environment and send a signal to the control center, which generates a response that is signaled to an effector. During the adaptation and feedback, the body expresses symptomatic changes such as inflammation and allergic reactions. Once the adaptation has settled down, the body begins to control the new homeostatic balance. Homeostasis is controlled by the nervous and endocrine systems in our body.

The hypothalamic regulation of anterior pituitary hormonal synthesis and release is integral to the regulation of stress, reproduction, metabolism, growth, and lactation. In brief, the integral function and target hormones are as follows:

- Stress: Cortisol
- Basal metabolism: Thyroid hormones
- Growth: Insulin-like growth factor
- Reproduction: Gonadal steroids

Each system follows the hierarchical axis. The hypothalamic–pituitary target organ axes are dependent on parallel regulatory systems. These axes have considerable cross talk with one another and can interact at multiple levels. This means that the hypothalamus gathers the complex information from the environment and reacts based on balance. Imbalance can also have an effect on other systems. For example, if you have taken birth control pills for many years, your basal temperature can be changed and it can affect your thyroid hormone level. Or, during a stressful situation, when your elevated stress hormone feeds back to the brain, it affects the regulation of stress as well as reproductive hormone regulation.

Type S is involved with most major hormone regulatory systems that maintain homeostasis, even though it has not been within the normal range or status in the cyclic loop. Moreover, these processes have developed over a long time, and can affect body postural habits.

Most type S is accompanied with multiple types of body shapes, such as types M2 and P or types M3 and T due to the adaptation to the new environment in an anatomical and physiologic way.

Type S is usually from the long-term adaptation process of body homeostasis, but sometimes the sudden disruption or interferences can affect the symptoms. The possible variations of disruption in the metabolic homeostatic cycle are hormone therapy, chemotherapy, sudden shock, intense emotional trauma, accidents, or surgery.

Lipedema

Most type S people are concerned about the fat deposits on their thighs, arms, hips, and lower legs, as lipedema starts on the lower extremities and upper arms. It results from lymph edema. If lymph edema is not resolved, skin flexibility is lost and expands with peripheral blood pressure, which is painful to touch or when applying exterior pressure. Lipedema is a long-term (chronic) condition typically involving an abnormal buildup of fat cells in the legs, thighs, and buttocks.

The condition occurs almost exclusively in women, although there have been rare cases reported in men, because woman have a special body fluids cycle. The woman's menstrual cycle affects her body's entire hormonal systems. Estrogen acts on osmotic regulation of arginine vasopressin (AVP), antidiuretic hormone (ADH), and body fluids.

In my clinical experience, patients with lipedema have a disturbed metabolic system (digestive issues may have been a problem for a long time), are taking hormonal medication, and are highly stressed, whether physically or mentally. More than two hormone disturbances are shown at the same time. The postural misalignment has occurred and pain symptoms are the main complaint.

Lipedema is not a single phenomenon in local fat deposition or congestion. It is involved with skin weakness, peripheral blood vessel pressure, subcutaneous congestion and scarring, muscle tightness, stretched tendon, and bone structure misalignment with metabolic homeostasis imbalances. This appearance affects physical activity and leads to emotional depression.

I have treated this condition as a sequential treatment plan based on major homeostatic balance. The systemic whole-body treatments help the circulation, breathing, and temperature, and reduce local congestion and excretions.

Pain

Mechanical Joint Pain

Most joint pain is related to the sympathetic nervous system, and the pain nerve is directly connected to the central nervous system. Except in the case of external traumas, joint pain is expected with muscles and tendon and ligament alignments. Chronic contracted muscles add stress to tendons and limit the range of motion, which results in poor circulation and misaligned bone structures.

Once the joint has been affected by failure to repair joint damage, it is diagnosed as osteoarthritis, a degenerative disorder breaking down cartilage and bone, leading to symptoms of pain, stiffness, and functional disability. The joint is surrounded by muscles, blood vessels, nerves, bursa, and soft tissues. Usually, joint movements are decided by the bone connecting muscles such as the biceps, and gastrocnemius. If muscles tighten, joint motion is limited. The limitation of motion results in poor circulation and congestion in the area. Poor circulation results in weakness of immune functions. It makes the joint area skin and other tissues sensitive to pathogens.

These processing of ailments has been observed and explained as bi syndrome in traditional Chinese medicine. Joint pain, a characteristic of bi syndrome, is caused by obstruction of Qi and blood in meridians and collaterals—due to invasion of pathogenic wind, cold, and damp. Furthermore, bi syndrome has a close relationship with the weather, body constitution, and skin defensive conditions. There are four major different syndromes according to symptoms and etiology: wind bi, cold bi, damp bi, and heat bi.

Chronic swelling on the body and heavy weight strain the joints, which can generate widespread pain through spinal pain receptors. Knee pain and ankle pain are common symptoms in type S. For preventing tightness of joint area, mild movement and a gentle range of motion are recommended, as well as the relaxation of muscle and tendons.

84 • *Body Reshaping through Muscle and Skin Meridian Therapy*

Metabolic Joint Pain

Another joint pain, such as gout, is possible in type S. Gout often accompanies metabolic syndrome, so it is known as metabolic joint pain. It is usually found in male patients and postmenopausal women. Gout, or monosodium urate crystal deposition disease, is the most common inflammatory arthritis. Uric acid is the by-product of purine metabolism in humans. Hyperuricemia predisposes affected persons to urate crystal formation and deposition, which lead to the inflammatory responses underlying the symptoms of gout.

Risk factors for hyperuricemia include obesity, hypertension, hyperlipidemia, insulin resistance, renal insufficiency, and use of diuretics. Diets rich in certain foods are also associated with increased risk for gout. Although gout symptoms show as a heat sign, high-quality moxa is used as the treatment method. Because most metabolic syndromes depend on blood circulation and volume, the severe pain and inflammatory heat signs are due to a delay in the circulation of Qi and blood in the meridians and collaterals caused by excessive cold. Moreover, cold causes the stagnation of blood and aggravates the pain.

In my experience, only the high quality of moxa can reduce the symptoms of gout with a broad treatment throughout the body's circulation and respiration.

POSTURAL CHARACTERISTICS

Type S posture is adapted on a chronic misaligned formation, and it is hard to detect the problem spot, as the swelling or congestion of the problem area has been covered several times with inflammatory reactions.

The body looks overweight or obese, either in localized areas or throughout the entire body.

Possible Associated Disorders

- Cushing syndrome
- Hypothyroidism or hyperthyroidism
- Polycystic ovarian syndrome (PCOS)
- Metabolic syndrome
- Infertility
- Premenstrual syndrome (PMS)
- Depression

Treatment

For type S treatment, the regulation of habit is based on periods such as bedtime, breakfast time, bath time, and skipping dinner. The time schedule control is recommended for at least six months to one year. In the clinic, skin treatment is the first step for relaxing body tension and regulating the body's thermostat. The second is focusing to clear the congestion, followed by skin treatments. It includes treatment of stretch marks, muscle tension, and body wrinkles.

During the treatment periods, type P and type T symptoms are shown alternatively. Especially, bloating and heaviness in the digestive system and allergic reaction may have occurred several times. When the other types of symptoms are shown, the treatment will be added for the symptoms.

The treatment rule is that if a pressure symptom is present, heat will be applied. If heat or cold signs are present, the pressure treatment will be chosen for types P and T.

Once the skin condition is better and even, the eight extraordinary meridians treatment can be applied to the treatment plan. The Dai channel and yang linking channel are prior to the Ren and Du channels.

Most type S patients need more time than other types of patients and have a slow body response. Some patients give up after several months, but some continue to see slow improvements.

For type S, patience and endurance are the most important steps for long-term planning of treatment.

Simple Home Therapy and Caution

Simplify Daily Life

Choose three important tasks according to stress level, such as work, commuting, chores, picking up children, and sleep. Once you know which ones are stressful and which are relaxing, you need to focus to do each level. If you are stressed at work and work hard, then your home should be a relaxing place and you need to focus on relaxing. Do not be distracted by others' drama or gossip and be bold in your time management.

Soften Your Body

Sometimes it is difficult to soften the body, but here are some tips:

1. Hum your favorite song with your mouth closed.
2. Count numbers with your fingers: Left to right fingers, count 1–10, and 10–1 right to left.
3. Once you are done finger counting, count numbers with a gentle wiggling motion of your toes.
4. You do not need to use big actions or stretch the ankle. Just feel your toes and continue to count left to right 1–10 and 10–1 right to left.
5. Then you will find that you are breathing deeply.

Keep Your Body Warm

You feel easily stuffy and hot, especially in the upper chest and head area, and are frequently thirsty and crave a cold drink. That is local congestion heat symptoms, which means the other parts of body temperature will be different than those of the congestion area. Before you drink cold water, or take off your clothes, check your ankle, knee, lower back, or abdomen with your hand and compare it with the chest or neck area with the other hand. You will probably feel the difference between the two hands, and then try to softly rub on the colder area for a while. It will get warmer soon. Then you can drink room temperature water instead of cold water.

Case Study

This case study involves a 36-year-old female whose main complaints (July 2013) were being overweight and lower back pain.

Brief History

The patient had been visiting my clinic since 2013 and was still not within the normal weight range on standard health charts. We tried to check her body mass index (BMI), but my machine could not detect her body mass index within its range.

Since outer appearance was not dramatically changed, nor did she look slimmer, her internal and external body functions and appearance were progressing positively. She had a large body since her youth, but she did not suffer from obesity. Almost five years ago, she suffered severe digestive problems, including painful bloating and diarrhea following an infection. Her stool cultures showed an intestinal problem from enterobacteria overgrowth. Her homeopathic doctor prescribed homeopathic antibiotics for 60 days. After that, her symptoms were relieved but her digestive system seemed weaker than before.

She traveled to southern Asia for several weeks and had severe cold symptoms during the trip. After returning home, she felt unwell and experienced digestive issues. She noticed that her abdominal area was enlarged and was still getting larger. She felt as though she were heavier each day. This was accompanied by lower back pain and knee pain. She tried to exercise and diet, but it aggravated her leg pain and back pain.

She visited several doctors for blood tests, was diagnosed as having a thyroid problem, and medication was prescribed. Several alternative practitioners recommended nutritional supplements and vitamins. A therapist prescribed antidepressant medications. She took the cocktail of pills. She enjoyed drinking alcohol in social settings and just for fun. She worked as a client services manager. During the weekend, she visited her family and slept on the couch.

She talked and laughed far more than is usual.

Observations

She looked tense and her whole body felt tight, and she seemed emotionally tight. During the initial sessions, she talked and laughed constantly with her friend. When I checked her skin, she had a fussy manner and was irritated. She almost shouted from pain when I applied gentle pressure. It was difficult for me to observe and palpate. Her body had lipedema on her arms and lower back to legs, and especially the side of the hip and thigh area had large fat deposits. Unlike ordinary lipedema, her condition showed extreme tension on the stretched skin area. That is why she could not tolerate touching. On the back of her leg and inner side were bulging veins and spider veins, and the ankle and dorsum of the feet were swollen like balloons.

Her abdomen had similar patterns. Both lower and upper fatty tissue deposits on the skin area were tense and seemed as though the outer shell was ballooning, which prevented palpation of the internal organ system. Her rib cage and shoulder were raised, and it was hard to palpate her neck because the shoulder area congestion was covered neck and face. The right-side rib cage had some deformed shape compared with the left side. It looked bigger and protruded. When I tried to push lightly, she felt severe pain on the liver area. Her skin was dry, but she had acne on her face and neck area. Her legs felt colder than other body parts and were X shaped, and she had flat feet.

Treatment Plan and Assessment

Her conditions represented type S, including types P and M2. She had been struggling for the previous five years and took several effective hormonal medications. She clearly shows the tension type of symptoms. Her leg shape, raised rib cage, and lower back pain indicate type M2.

It is thus important to explain the treatment duration for type S and possible side effects during the treatments. For example, she had a lipedema condition underneath skin tension; once the tension was reduced, what remained was uneven, bumpy skin that had expanded but was not flexible enough to shrink as the tension beneath decreased, and it appeared as though the area beneath the loose skin was waterlogged. This is when people think that the situation has become worse or there was extra weight gain. However, the treatment can be continued and improve skin tightness and peripheral blood vessel dilation, remove extracellular water, and so forth.

As she had tension and pressure symptoms, treatment was started with hyperthermal therapy and GIR for reducing the tension on the abdominal area for breathing and circulation. For several sessions, only her abdominal area was treated with heat methods. Body fluid drops appearing as a sweating condition indicated that the tension was being released. After releasing the abdominal tension, the breathing muscle was treated with muscle meridian acupuncture techniques.

In the meantime, she was recommended a half-body bath, soaking only the lower abdominal area, and waiting until her forehead began sweating. She was also recommended to keep the ankle area protected with a comfortable pressure band. This is for ankle blood pump facilitation.

Instead of vigorous exercise, she tried to move her ankles and feet gently and slowly while lying down and during bath time for daily exercise. Her multiple cocktail supplements were stopped, except the thyroid medication, which was prescribed by a medical doctor. She stopped drinking alcohol. Subsequently, she stopped the thyroid medication at the end of spring 2015.

Now we are working on postural correction in the torso area. She still looks big and has not much changed her outlook, but I can palpate her ribs, abdominal muscles, and hip muscles individually. Her back pain is reduced and her spinal condition better, which can be seen in the separation between the neck and shoulder. When I touch her skin, she no longer complains, and the acne has cleared.

During the last two years, she was promoted at work and traveled on several occasions. She has progressed well and is ailment-free, without the use of any medication. Most of all, she is confident about her health and now manages her condition.

6

Anatomical Approach:
Types M1, M2, and M3

TYPE M1 (FIGURE 6.1)

Quick Tips

1. Open the hands and spread the fingers wide apart and hold that position firmly. Then slowly roll your head in a circular motion about your shoulders while your palm and fingers remain widely spread apart. If you feel uncomfortable and experience some pain, your symptoms include type M1 yang.
2. Make a fist with both hands and hold firmly, then breathe; inhale and exhale. Next, relax your hands and fingers as much possible, then wave your hands gently, and breathe at the same time. Compare the two different motions and breathing, and if you find breathing much easier while waving your hands, then you are probably close to type M1 yin.

Related Condition

Please check if you have these symptoms:

- Frequent sinus infection and runny nose, puffiness under the eyes, earache, or ear infection
- Feeling tired and fatigued, want to eat or drink frequently even when not hungry or thirsty, bloating easily, especially in the upper abdomen right after eating
- Shoulder pain and upper back pain; sometimes forearm tension and finger stiffness
- Fatty tissue deposit on the back side of arms and armpits, swollen feeling in breast area, and fat accumulation on the side of the rib cage
- Sad feeling but not depressed, more anxiety, hurried and worried

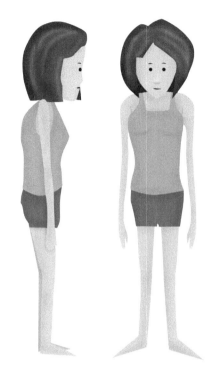

FIGURE 6.1
Type M1.

- Facial skin trouble, hair loss, dry skin, discoloration of skin on upper neck and arm area
- Indecisive and lack of self-confidence
- Have a history of surgery on the upper body area, such as the thorax, upper back, neck, arm, shoulder, and face

Clinical Syndrome

Type M1 patients usually complain of pain in the shoulders and neck, tension headaches, allergic symptoms (runny nose, itchy eyelids, sore throat, etc.), anxiety and depression, and general feeling of sadness. These symptoms are similar to those experienced in type P; however, type P involves more complicated physiologic problems than type M1.

In type P, neck and arm muscles are prominent and classified as diagnosis clues. For type M1, when lying on the abdomen, the neck area shows horizontal wrinkles, but type P tends to be more swollen and with a round neck and shoulder and tension in the upper back (Figure 6.2).

Type M1 presents with upper extremity discomfort and problems such as arm pain, arm weakness, wrist pain, rheumatoid arthritis pain, finger joint pain, and finger gout.

There are two different subtypes, type M1 yang and type M1 yin. Most type M1 patients have both subsyndromes, but the progress of the disorder connection will follow a different direction. For diagnostic convenience in treatment, I have classified the subcategories. Type M1 yang usually originates from working with or partaking in activities that use hands in a pronated position, such as typing on a keyboard, driving, dental work, and design. Type M1 yin is usually caused by passive incidents, such as surgery, injury, trauma, accidents, and atrophy from chronic illness, inflammation, or infection. This condition is associated with lymphatic congestion and the breathing muscle group.

Understanding the Mechanism

Body movement is not merely a single motion. For instance, the distal fingertip or toe movement results in all connective muscles, fascia, bones, blood vessels, and lymphatic vessels moving simultaneously (Figure 6.3).

We can imagine how muscles work and support each other when we use the keyboard on a computer. At first, your arms should be in a forward position and your forearms pronate with flexion of your wrists. The motion needs to rotate the hand and arm inward. While rotating the hand and arm, the rotator cuff muscles are

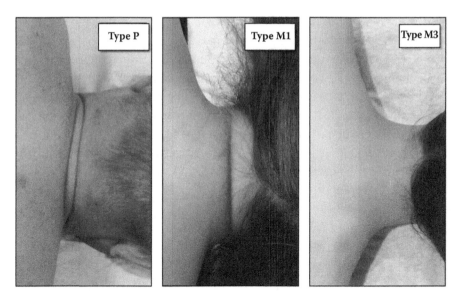

FIGURE 6.2
Neck wrinkle differentiation.

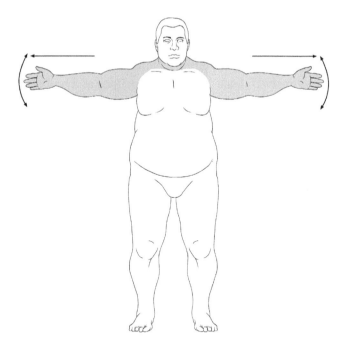

FIGURE 6.3
Type M1 mechanism.

engaged within the shoulder. For pronating forearms, two muscles, the pronator teres and pronator quadratus, work together by pulling on the radius bone of the forearm. The radius is rotated at the elbow and wrist joints around the other forearm bone, the ulna, which is supported on the desk to ease up and down movement of the fingers, and a bent wrist rests on the desk for horizontal movement. This action overworks the biceps and overextends the triceps. It also affects chest muscles by tightening them and pulls the shoulders forward. This position may be maintained all day if you work at a desk on a computer, take long car trips, have a career as a dentist, hairdresser, or cook, or work in a factory where you partake in repetitive motion.

Pain and posture problems are not always caused by skilled or repetitive work, but symptoms of bad posture may present themselves if a balanced condition and environment is disturbed by regular life. Usually the pain is the primary concern for patients, and practitioners can help them determine the pathologic progression.

Muscles need several aiding muscle groups when being used or maintaining a certain posture. If you have a local or referred pain on your shoulder or back, you should be aware of the movement involved or which muscles are involved. Even if it is a minor finger motion, the finger to shoulder and head areas work together and influence each other. This will better aid in understanding and calculating the motion involved. Movement in the distal part of the body employs the aid of more muscles and joints; even skin and tissue are involved and have an effect, depending on the connection. That is why muscle and sinew meridians form part of the diagnosis, treatment map, and guidelines.

The muscle and sinew meridians are introduced in Chapter 7. Since type M1 yang syndrome focuses on active and passive muscles, the myofascial treatments are effectively applied with acupuncture, trigger points, massage, and other myofascial-targeted treatment methods.

However, myofascial treatments are not as effective in type M1 yin syndrome, because the posture change or muscle tensions of type M1 yin are due mostly to breathing muscle contractions or armpit lymphatic congestions. Even though the pain sensation is in the same or a similar region as type M1 yang, the etiology is different. Subjectively, patients have more upper back and side fat in type M1 yin, whereas the upper shoulder, neck, facial swelling, and fat are present in type M1 yang.

Pain

In clinical observation and treatment, the type M1 group of patients complain of major shoulder and upper back pain. The pain generates mostly from the upper thorax, and the pain experienced is commonly a referred pain sensation. Often, the source of the pain cannot be recognized due to peripheral sensory nerve damage. However, pain can be communicated through facial expressions and bodily movements.

When meeting with a traditional Chinese medicine (TCM) practitioner, you will be asked about the quality of the pain, such as distending pain, pulling, sharp, dull, cold sensation with pain, and burning pain, because the etiology of pain varies vastly. Then the actual pain area will be palpated with a finger or hand to make an objective diagnosis. Some areas feel good when pressure is applied, while some do not.

Pain qualities are distinguished by three different levels in a medical examination. The first category is the paroxysmal extreme pain sensations, such as shooting, sharp, electric, hot, and radiating. The second category is the superficial pain, such as itchy, cold, numb, sensitive, and tingling. The third category is deep pain, including aching, heavy, dull, cramping, and throbbing.

Myofascial pain is more typical of type M1, whereas the quality of pain in type P is somewhat different. In comparison, neck pain in type M1 patients is typically more localized, while type P patients usually express tension in the neck and shoulder area or neck and headaches, especially after a large meal or drinking alcohol.

Muscle Connection and Function in Type M1

Shoulder protraction is a prominent posture characteristic of type M1. Shoulder protraction causes shortening of the sternomastoid muscle and draws the head anteriorly and inferiorly. It is possible to develop a deformity because of the adaptive shortening of scalene and pectoralis minor muscles. Such deformity also presents with a narrowed costoclavicular space (ribs 1–5 are relatively elevated). Other muscles, such as the trapezius, levator scapulae, and serratus anterior muscles, are also involved. The most commonly involved are the trapezius and the levator scapulae region.

The condition of the upper back muscles changes due to eccentric contraction. This repetitive action causes sequential tendinomuscular degeneration. However, in healthy people, skeletal muscle degeneration is usually accompanied by regeneration responding to the trigger of inflammation. However, since inflammation causes pain, it delays the muscle functions and contributes to fibrosis, which is usually found at the intersection point of two or more muscles.

On the other hand, type M1 yin syndrome originates from local circulatory congestions, especially on the root from the torso and arms. One of my patients had a childhood trauma, a left arm dislocation; she avoided using her left arm since the incident, and she did not have many symptoms until she visited my clinic. Her main complaint was shoulder pain and neck pain, but she also expressed the desire to reduce her breast size and sought the advice of a plastic surgeon even though her breast size was not above average and should not have caused discomfort. She experienced excessive pressure and a general feeling of discomfort in her breast area.

This case of sequential deformity followed the trauma that occurred. Pain and weakness, scar tissue, chronic tendonitis, and lymphatic congestion chronically occurred because of the process of regeneration. The medial arm line to the armpit and chest area was affected by the circulatory system reaction due to the trauma. Side congestion caused the shoulder adduction muscle group to become weakened. Because restricted mobility is usually accompanied by congestion, and vice versa, the congestion results in a range of motion limitation.

The shoulder adduction muscle group includes the pectoralis major, subscapularis, teres major, latissimus dorsi, and coracobrachialis. In my experiences, when type M1 yin treatment is focused on treating the armpit wrinkle line and the shoulder adduction muscles, the result is more effective.

Postural Characteristics

- Face: Facial asymmetric conditions such as wrinkles on one side, masseter muscle asymmetrical contraction, and acne or skin trouble on one side.
- Neck: Wrinkles and fat accumulation on the back of the neck; the length of the neck is different in the front and back.
- Arms: When in a natural standing posture, the dorsum of the hand can be seen while making a fist.

- Hand and fingers: Stiff feeling with hand open and fingers widespread, or difficulty in closing fist due to forearm and upper arm muscle tightness.
- Clavicle: V shape, hard to distinguish the clavicle bone.
- Skin: T1–T7 (thoracic spine 1–7) area discoloration, back part of deltoid area discoloration, occiput area psoriasis-like skin eruption or discoloration, acne on upper back and lower chin area.
- Blood vessels: Jugular, hand, and arm veins prominent.
- Range of motion: Arm supine position difficulty, limitation in raising arm, hunchback posture.
- Spine: Hunched back, upper thoracic but shoulder raised, square shoulder shape.
- Behavior: Shortness of breath, shallow breathing, anxiety and sadness, want quick results.
- If patient lies down, the rib cage looks wide and intercostal space is narrow.

Possible Associated Disorders

- Temporomandibular joint (TMJ) disorder: Grinding teeth, migraine headache without aura, temporal vein prominent
- Thoracic outlet syndrome
- Tendonitis
- Myofascial pain
- Arthritis
- Bursitis
- Torticollis
- Winged scapulae

Following the hand yang meridian muscle channel (eccentric contraction with chronic lymph congestion), we can find stretch marks and goose bump–shaped fat deposit skin eruptions. For the hand yin meridian muscle channel, muscle and fascia tension is located alongside the palm, forearm, cubitus, armpit, and side chest between the arm and torso. The muscle meridian treatment starts at the distal to the proximal of the body. Check the hand motions.

Simple Home Therapy and Caution

- Relax the shoulder and entire arm, and then try to rotate your wrist in a circular motion.
- In a lying-down position, arms relaxed with palm upside, curl the fingers slowly and gently until the wrist curls.
- Frequently check your arm and chest area.
- During a shower or bath, scrub your body along the finger-to-torso and finger-to-face line.

Case Study

This case study involves a 35-year-old female.

Brief History

A 35-year-old female attended my clinic on February 21, 2013, and expressed her desire to begin a weight loss program, the "reset detox diet" program. She wanted to lose weight quickly and seemed depressed and anxious. The patient worked in a financial company as a manager and spent all day at a desk using a computer.

Her posture was forward inclined with a noticeable waist and arm line. Her hip muscle appeared very weak and her trousers did not fit her waistline. Her legs were X shaped and her arms in a pronate position while standing. Her shoulders protruded and her neck was straight, but the sternocleidomastoid muscle (SCM) was tight. Her skin and facial complexion were dark, and facial acne scars were prominent on both the cheeks and forehead. She reported having had severe acne even before puberty.

She mentioned that her poor posture was an adjustment to playing with normal-height friends in elementary school because she was the tallest child at school; as a result, she hunched her upper back. She did not take any medication, but sometimes took painkillers to treat severe shoulder and neck pain. Her digestion was good, but she admitted to eating too much and wanted to control her appetite.

Her weight loss target areas were upper arms, "love handles," and thighs. Since she was not satisfied with her body, she had tried various diets for weight loss, including juicing, low-fat diets, low-carbohydrate diets, fasting diets, and exercise. While the dieting was helpful for temporarily losing weight, once she went to back to her normal diet, she regained weight.

Her daily lifestyle consisted of a 9:00 a.m.–6:00 p.m. workday with a one-hour lunch break, and her schedule did not allow for daily exercise. Her challenge was maintaining a healthy diet and regular exercise while working for a company where business trips and time zone changes especially disturbed her body balance. For these reasons, she had tried a repetitive diet plan but felt unhealthy, both physically and mentally. This made her feel depressed and despondent.

Her menstrual cycle was irregular and she suffered from acne during menstruation. She also suffers from dysmenorrhea and premenstrual syndrome. She often gave in to comfort eating and consumed excessive amounts of food.

Observations

Her body shape was a typical type M1, and her upper thoracic area appeared forward inclined and her SCM was shortened and fixed. Her chin was pulled downward. Her shoulders and arms protruded and displayed tension toward the medial aspect. There was clear evidence of hypercurvature of the cervical spine and tension of SCM under her ears. Examination of her eyes and sinuses revealed swelling and congestion.

The patient's rear-side deltoid muscles were weak, large, and flabby with evidence of water congestion with tension. Her rib cage protruded, was rounded, and inclined upward, which necessitated palpation on the first rib while the patient was supine in a lying-down position. The sternum was raised on the third and fourth ribs and her clavicle was narrowed and V shaped.

Her lower abdomen had tension and fatty tissue congestion. The gluteus was weak and the pelvis was tilted anteriorly. Examination of her legs revealed several small bruised areas, an indication that she bruised easily on her legs. There were also signs of chronic toe infection and her leg muscle tone was weak, with stretched (lengthened) contraction on the thigh area, but swelling without tension. The abdominal area displayed the greatest signs of tension, but all extremities were loose.

There was no indication of allergic reactions, and the patient did not mention any either.

For the digestive system, her upper middle area was hard (like pressing on cheesecake) and a gentle push made her feel uncomfortable. The umbilical region was soft at first and then hardened. Overall, the abdomen had internal peritoneum tension.

Her arms were in the pronate posture and she complained of pain and discomfort when attempting to change to a supine position. The back of the arms and armpit area indicated lymphatic water congestion without tension. The area was discolored and darker than other areas. The skin of the congested area was loose and presented with irregular stretch marks.

The muscle tone of her arms was weak, and the biceps and triceps felt stringlike when palpated; the biceps were shortened but small, thick, and stringy, whereas the triceps presented as thin and long, stringlike shapes. The scapulae protruded and were raised almost 45°; the levator scapulae, located on the uppermost shoulder, were very tight and difficult to palpate. The rotator cuff muscles were tight, and a knot structure was discovered beneath the discolored skin.

Examination of the spine showed that the thoracic 2 to lumbar spines were straightened and her back muscles were very tight, but as the skin was dry and swollen, it was difficult to distinguish between the spine and spinal muscle area. The sacral area and coccyx were depressed and gluteus muscles were loose and weak. The patient's legs were X shaped even when she lay on her abdomen. The gastrocnemius and soleus could not be separated and muscle tone was poor. The ankle vein was prominent, swollen, and averted.

The skin of the patient was discolored and varied in quality. Her extremities were all dry, loose, and flabby. The armpit, inguinal lymph area, and side of the torso area were dark with prominent sweat pores.

Assessment and Plan (Treatment Plan)

Subjective and objective assessments showed that there were type M1, M3, and P symptoms and signs that were complicated, and a change in habits was needed. Type P has several different types manifested in the area presenting with tension. In this patient, her extremities were depressed and her torso pressed.

Dark skin and abdominal tension indicated that chronic pain or discomfort was caused by a misaligned posture and irregular eating habits. Even though her case involved many symptoms and signs that needed to be treated and corrected, the priority of the plan was for long-term maintenance, even after treatment had been covered.

Discussion Regarding Plans and Treatment Order Each Week

Since her type P condition is categorized as the "body trunk pressed and extremities depressed." This case treatment is effective in dealing with tension areas. She had tension in her abdomen and face, but when treating abdominal tension, we treat the corresponding back area first. Patients with abdominal tension experience lower or middle back pain because the front and back are not separable. One side is pulling and the other is being pulled. The area between the pulling and that which is being pulled is folded. In this case, the abdomen was pulling, the lower back was being pulled, and the body was being folded.

So, before treating the pulling, I was required to make certain exactly what the pulled and the folded were. This can be applied to any condition, but usually the pulled area is a tendon, ligament, or fascia level that is not very flexible. It is important to check the skin temperature. If it is cold, the approach is to apply moxa oil or moxa with heat and apply moving cupping toward the folded area. The folded area may have stretch marks or fluid congestion, which is fatty tissue. If the skin displays heat symptoms, I would omit the moxa oil and moxa and only apply cupping on the folded area.

Gastrointestinal resuscitation (GIR) is the best treatment for type P torso tension. The basic components of GIR are warming, gentle pressure, and gentle movement on the abdomen. Usually the medium is an indirect moxa cone, but I recently opted to use moxa hand oil. Once GIR is complete, patients feel relieved and comfortable; some have a sleepy and tired sensation. There are many ways to manipulate the abdomen, such as abdominal massage, gastrointestinal manipulation, and acupressure.

Once GIR is completed, a hyperthermal tool should be applied to the abdomen. An infrared heat lamp, infrared dome, or moxa heating pad can be found in most acupuncture clinics. Otherwise, one would put a blanket on the manipulated area to keep it warm.

Postural imbalance caused pain in the patient's lower back and shoulders. The hand yang meridian and foot yin meridian treatment were selected, because the order of muscle meridian treatment commences on the weaker part of body. Type M1's weak meridian is the hand 3 yang meridian, and type M3's weak meridian is the foot 3 yin meridian. The muscle meridian acupuncture technique is used in weak muscle meridians, piercing the wrinkle line with a 0.16 needle gauge, and manipulating in three to eight directions.

Moxa oil gua sha treatment is used in an antagonistic strong muscle meridian; apply moxa oil with a tongue depressor or gua sha tool on the targeted line and gently scrape, following the muscle meridian line. After using the gua sha tool, red dots may be visible along the meridian. The intensity of the redness will depend on the condition of peripheral blood vessel congestion, lymphatic congestion, or muscle tightness. Usually, extreme pain may be experienced due to lymphatic congestion, even though the practitioner takes care in ensuring the problem area is scraped very gently.

I recommended that the patient eat and sleep on a regular basis, and before going to bed, it was advised that she take a half-body bath. Understanding nutrition, what our bodies need, and how they work is an important health education subject. Her diet pattern had been focused on her weight gain and calorie calculations. Each week we focused on a new health issue and observed the implementation of changes and outcomes together. Great emphasis was placed on discussing the way that her body changed after treatment and the use of home remedies.

Results

The patient commenced treatment in February 2013. She still visits regularly in order to maintain her health. In the interim, her lower back and shoulder pain have been alleviated. Her poor neck posture was corrected, and as a result, her face is less puffy and her complexion looks brighter and smoother. Her digestive system is no longer a concern. She is happier and more confident, and is now more objective about the emotions that she allows herself to feel and is able to choose which emotions rule her life. She is also more secure about her emotional status.

Her emotional stability and positive attitude have improved her lifestyle; she was confident enough to negotiate a promotion, take on new hobbies, and enjoy better relationships with friends and coworkers. Improved physical health allowed her to take control of her mind, and so she overcame burdens and difficulties more easily. Now she plays golf and walks every day, not for weight loss, but for sheer enjoyment. She no longer needs to concern herself with the number on the scale, because she can palpate her waistline and her inner joy is reflected in the mirror. She bakes cookies and shares them with friends. She enjoys and appreciates food and meals, without counting calories and being concerned with nutritional factors or worrying about weight gain. She understands that a healthy digestive system can absorb and excrete, rather than blaming the food she eats or feeling guilty after a meal.

Health is hard to define in one word. According to the World Health Organization (WHO) health concept, food is "a resource for everyday life, not the objective of living. Health is a positive concept emphasizing social and personal resources, as well as physical capacities." The patient is free from pain, and this is an influential factor in her newfound quality of life. Her ability to take care of herself has had a positive effect on her daily life. She is involved with and takes pride in performing her job and social activities.

An overall body-reshaping program is the educational medium to transfer to individual health through the experience of positive physical change.

TYPE M2 (FIGURE 6.4)

Quick Tips

1. If you lie down on a hard floor, the full supine posture (lying face up) will be uncomfortable for the type M2 group.

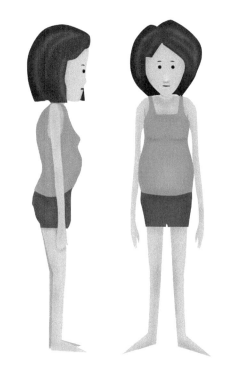

FIGURE 6.4
Type M2.

Then try to switch to a semisupine position, lying on your back, bending your knees, and putting your feet on the floor. This position should be much more comfortable and relaxing.

2. Once you are lying down, find your side waistline. Simply place your hand on your lower back and move toward the side and front following the waistline. If you notice the side of your waist is bigger than your hip and upper abdomen, you are categorized as type M2.

3. Again, while you are lying down in a supine position, palpate your upper abdomen around your bony rib area; you will probably notice your rib cage is protruding or the angle of your rib cage is larger than 90°.

4. Breathe deeply, especially while trying to focus on your inhalation. If you

find it somewhat difficult to inhale, then raise your arms and inhale and exhale. Much easier? Now consider, why do you raise your arms while riding a rollercoaster in an amusement park?

Related Condition

- Heartburn, bloating, indigestion
- Sleep disorder (eating before bedtime aids in a good night's sleep)
- Weight concerns (abdominal area)
- Difficulty in controlling eating habits
- Love handles, "muffin top"
- Lower back and shoulder pain
- Fat deposits under the armpit and on the side of your body
- Fatigue and easily tired
- Emotional (easily angered and easily depressed)
- Sitting position preferred over standing and running
- Frontal headache, nose congestion, sinus infection
- Stretch marks on belly button area

Clinical Syndrome

Type M2 can often be undistinguishable from types M1 and M3, as it has very similar patterns.

Unlike types M1 and M3, type M2 has symptoms and signs of the upper thorax, neck, and lower pelvic girdle area, simultaneously. The component problem of type M1 only radiates to each side of the breathing muscles and facial muscles. A type M3 disorder begins in the pelvic area, moving toward the midspine and back of the head. However, disorders associated with type M2 can affect the entire body, especially the outer shell, for example, sudden weight gain

of the whole body, general body pains without inflammation or infection, and emotional outbursts.

Noticeable body shapes such as a protruding rib cage, a palpable mass under the xiphoidal process, the angle of the xiphoid, and spine lordosis with weakness of the iliocostalis lumborum are useful diagnostic pillars.

Type M2 has been nicknamed the "pregnant woman shape" and "sway back," due to the presence of lordosis, which is an exaggerated lumbar curvature. This condition is caused by an overdeveloped or shortened latissimus dorsi, lower erector spinae, hip flexors, and lengthening of the rectus abdominis and hip extensors.

Sitting on a chair for long periods has been criticized by many posture-concerned practitioners. Because the hip flexion posture is similar to that of a sitting posture, patients' complaints of lower back pain and knee pain help rule out disorder of the hip flexor muscle group. Many therapists and trainers focus on stretching the hip flexor muscle group and strengthening abdominal muscles. This approach is beneficial for some people. However, my clinical approach to lower back pain and a protruding abdomen differs from most theories.

Abdominal muscle tightness is not ideal, as these muscles support and cover the abdominal cavity and connect the rib cage. Breathing and diaphragmatic actions are indirectly influenced by the abdominal cavity fluid balance and peristaltic movement. Furthermore, the function of abdominal muscles includes flexion, lateral bending, and circular rotation with the myofascial netting structures. The different direction of each abdominal muscle and aponeurosis can allow for regulation of internal pressure and multidirectional, free movement. This unique structure can help tighten the circular abdominal cavity and, at the same time, aid breathing.

I focus on loosening the abdominal muscles so that movement while inhaling and exhaling can be observed. Unlike other skeletal muscles, strengthened abdominal muscles should center on increased flexibility and mobility; imagine the free movements of belly dancers and hula dancers. Therefore, it is understandable that dynamic and active digestive viscera will prefer free movement, such as that of a hammock, opposed to a hard metal surface, not allowing for much movement.

Many female patients experience type M2 syndrome, especially after childbirth. They complain of multiple issues simultaneously, mostly pain and digestive issues. The reduction of abdominal obesity is the focus in type M2 patients, regardless of whether they appear slim.

Type M2 lordosis concerns are usually accompanied by abdominal bloating or a distinctive ballooning shape. In the case of liver dysfunction, the ballooning shape of the abdomen results in lower back pain. Both cases are present when the diaphragm is strained and the breathing muscles contracted. Excess abdominal congestion may affect breathing by pressing on the diaphragm and chest wall, making it harder for the lungs to fill with air. Allergic reactions and coughing are common symptoms of type M2.

Uncomfortable breathing and bloating may cause emotional disturbances such as anxiety and depression. Individuals in the type M2 group tend to alternately experience opposite feelings. It is not sadness or grief, but more like anxiety and depression, so I have nicknamed it the "pressed and depressed type."

Sitting or standing for long periods of time, or even pregnancy, causes swelling in the legs, especially in the ankle area. A lack of ankle flexibility may affect posture and muscle tension. Lower extremity disorders result from a lack of activity, and a sedentary lifestyle may result in lower extremity disorders. For type M2 patients, flexibility in the ankle region is very important.

Understanding the Mechanism

Type M2 affects full body flexibility, especially the outer shell in the front, side, and back vertically, while type M1 targets the left tips of the fingers to the right sides of the fingertips across the upper chest area horizontally (Figure 6.5). The body has sagittal frame structures, such as the chest diaphragm and pelvic diaphragm, with vertical frames including front, back, and sides. Sagittal frames surround and connect with vertical frames.

Any motion (action, sitting, standing, and sleeping) and posture depend on gravity. Every object has a center of gravity located at the point where an object can be perfectly balanced, and so too, the human body has a center of gravity. The center of gravity in the human body is an anatomical position found approximately in the middle of the sacrum. When walking or bending, the center of gravity will move and be adapted to the situation and environment.

Sudden changes to the body, such as pregnancy, can effect a change in the center of gravity, but the body can afford to adapt to these balance changes for nine months. However, long-term changes result in an unnatural posture and so cause abdominal obesity.

However, the real structural concern is that of the outer shell connections that are

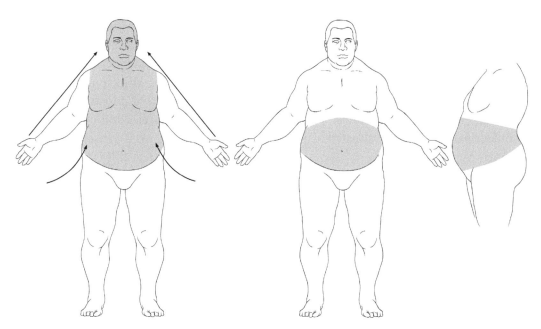

FIGURE 6.5
Type M2 mechanism.

contracted or lengthened, or stretched muscles, ligaments, tendons, skin, and soft tissues. They support and preserve the center of gravity. Type M2 disorders display deformities of the outer structure of the chest diaphragm and pelvic diaphragm. Imagine the body as a flexible accordion with a cylindrical shape, and the area between the two cross sections being pushed outward due to internal pressure. The stretched side will have tension and the contracted side will have wrinkles.

If you want to even out the cylindrical shape, you will need to lengthen it by holding the top and bottom of the cylinder to adjust its height. It will be very difficult to adjust the length by pushing on the middle section.

Type M2 Muscle Connections and Functions

In theory, many muscles are involved in a state of lordosis; the major role-playing muscles in type M2 are the latissimus dorsi muscle and hip flexors. Hip flexors are composed of the iliopsoas, iliacus, rectus femoris, and tensor fascia latae. The latissimus dorsi muscle originates from the spinous process of the lower six thoracic vertebrae, lumbar vertebrae, and sacral vertebrae; the iliac crest of the hip bone; and the lower three or four ribs. It finally attaches to the bottom of the intertubercular groove of the humerus.

Latissimus dorsi muscles cover the lower and midback and connect with the hip, spine, and upper arm, having an effect on the action of the arm. The latissimus dorsi also extends, adducts, and medially rotates the arm. It draws the shoulder downward and backward and keeps the inferior angle of the scapula against the chest wall. It therefore works as an antagonist of the deltoid and trapezius and aids in raising of the trunk above the arm. Hence, it is also called the climbing muscle. Since the latissimus dorsi muscle rotates the shoulder and depresses the shoulder girdle, it puts pressure on the brachial flexus, which is a nerve bundle running from the cervical spine into the arm, including the hand, and innervates these regions. This tension generates neck and shoulder pain. Sometimes, patients' shoulder pain has been mistreated by practitioners for this reason.

The important factor is that it winds around the lower border of the teres major muscle and forms posterior folds of axilla. The area will display the skin wrinkles or stretch marks, and depending on the condition and symptoms, this can be a good diagnosis and treatment guide.

The latissimus dorsi muscle is connected to the thoracolumbar fascia, which is covered by the iliocostalis, longissimus, multifidus, and quadratus lumborum muscles. The thoracolumbar fascia directly connects to the latissimus dorsi and outer shape of the transversus abdominis. It is also connected to the vertebral body. The connection between the latissimus dorsi and transversus abdominis and internal oblique muscles is the key to getting rid of love handles, also called a muffin top, which are excess fat deposits on the sides of the torso. Love handles can cause lower back pain and lipoma on the back if not treated. I treat this condition with the eight extraordinary channel systems.

The abdominal muscles are a unique structure, able to connect the upper rib cage and lower pelvis, and cover and support the abdominal cavity and its internal organs. The fibers of the three layers of muscle in the anterolateral wall provide maximum strength. The deepest layer is the transverse abdominis, which is connected with the lumbosacral fascia to the ribs and pelvis, compresses the abdomen, and rotates the trunk laterally with the external oblique

muscle. The area between the transverse abdominis and external oblique, the internal oblique muscle, connects the pelvis and lumbosacral fascia. This muscle has the important function of posture; it holds all the abdominal muscles and pulls the front of the pelvis upward. It causes the lumbar spinal curve to flatten. If it is not functioning correctly, the abdomen will protrude and spinal lordosis may develop.

Another muscle, the rectus abdominis, connects the sternum to the pubic symphysis, aids forced expiration, childbirth, and defecation, as well as compresses the abdominal cavity. Abdominal muscles are antagonist to the diaphragm, relaxing as it contracts. This is one of the major causes of sleep apnea. During sleep, the only active skeletal muscle is the diaphragm, which aids in breathing. If the abdominal muscles are too tight and have difficulty in relaxing, it has an effect on the diaphragm muscle action.

Since the latissimus dorsi muscle is connected to the lower three or four ribs, it assists in the breathing system. By raising your arms upward, you are able to ease inhalation difficulties. In TCM, the organ relationship theory mentions the breathing system: lung Qi controls respiration, and kidney Qi coordinates inhalation. Weakness of the lower back is typical of aging and one of the symptoms of kidney deficiency in TCM.

Type M2 is related to anterior pelvic tilt syndrome, which is caused by lumbar lordosis and thoracic kyphosis, stretched and tightened abdominal muscles, and tightened hip flexor muscles. It leads to lower back pain, hip pain, knee pain, and flat feet.

Type M2 disorders center around lordosis, abdominal tension, love handles, and so forth. The treatment approach covers the entire outer shell of the body, along the foot yang muscle tendon meridian, which runs along the foot to the head in all four dimensions (Figure 6.6).

Below is a summary for understanding the type M2 mechanism:

- The most dynamic change is to the abdominal area.
- The factors of change are abdominal cavity pressure or volume pushing out in all directions.
- The abdominal area is located between the chest diaphragm and pelvic diaphragm, which are influenced by internal pressure.
- The upper chest diaphragm affects the upper chest and back, and even the neck posture.
- The neck affects facial muscle expression.
- The lower pelvic diaphragm affects the pelvis, legs, and feet.

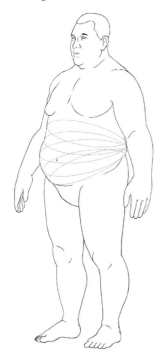

FIGURE 6.6
Type M2 outer shell mechanism.

Type M2 should be considered with a three-dimensional balancing aspect of diagnosis and treatment, which means that there is an equilibrium in tightening and lengthening. Only focusing on the two aspects (tightening and lengthening) will not be as successful.

Pain

Lower back, hip, and knee pain are common symptoms of type M2. An anterior pelvic tilt posture causes the hamstrings and hip muscles (gluteus muscles) to lengthen, and the antagonist muscles (quadriceps femoris and hip flexors) to shorten into a static posture. Once the quadriceps femoris muscles are tight, a bent knee will incline toward the medial and a flexed ankle toward the lateral side of the body. These actions will result in the knee and leg rotating inwardly and the foot will be overpronated. From a clinical aspect, misaligned legs present as hip bursitis, knee meniscus pain, a valgus knee shape, and flat feet due to hyperpronation subtalar inversion.

Type M2 lower back pain is accompanied by the accumulation of body fluids or tissues. If chronic back pain is not cleared, a line of soft or tight mass of fat can be noticed. Sometimes this mass, or lipoma, can be palpable. Pain in the lower back is not always due to muscle pain or nerve pain. Skin tightness and pressure must also be considered as a culprit of the pain.

Other common symptoms of type M2 are abdominal distension and bloating. Distension and bloating are rather different from each other, but sometimes present together. Clinically, they are related to functional gastrointestinal disorders (FGIDs) and motility disorders that include irritable bowel syndrome (IBS), functional dyspepsia, and chronic constipation. Both bloating and distension cause discomfort and pain. The symptoms may relate to frequent burping or belching, swallowing air, and passing intestinal gas.

Postural Characteristics

- Face: Vertical frowns between eyebrows.
- Neck: If type M1 is involved, neck posture will be that of the type M1 position; if only type M2 is present, a forward-inclined neck posture will be observed.
- Arm: Medial rotation with a kyphosis posture, although not severe, as the shoulders tend to be depressed; if severe, winged scapulae.
- Hands and fingers: Cold hands and feet, weak and numb, arthritic pain.
- Clavicle: Not prominent.
- Skin: Stretch marks on abdomen, horizontal dark lines on lower back.
- Blood vessels: Varicose veins and spider veins.
- Range of motion: Difficulty in rotation of the upper part of the trunk, shoulder adduction is not fully engaged.
- Spine: Lordosis, sway back, possible kyphosis, short torso, and long lower limbs.
- Legs: Knock-knees, valgus syndrome.
- Behavior: Emotional instability, anxiety and depression, laughing and speaking louder.

Possible Associated Disorders

- Postpartum depression
- Hepatic disorder
- Functional gastrointestinal disorders

Treatment

The foot yang muscle tendon meridians are used in the diagnosis and treatment plan of type M2. These meridians run from the toes to the head, covering the front, back, and side areas of the body. The first points of examination are the lumbosacral area, armpits, back of the knee, neck, and ankle structures. Then skin conditions are examined.

Once a treatment plan has been assessed, semicircular body treatments can be started. Semicircular body perspectives change the viewpoint of criteria as the body sectional connection from the spine to the frontal midline. This means that the basic position should be "lying on the side" and the midline is the middle of the side line. While a patient lies on his or her side, the spine to midline will be treated.

Body wrinkles are treated with acupuncture, and the flexion scraped with moxa oil and cupping.

Muscle meridian needling techniques are applied to the lengthened muscles and between the muscles starting on the anterior superior iliac spine (ASIS) area, while the patient's leg is pulled by a practitioner in the hip extension position. Following that, the latissimus dorsi muscle is treated in the armpit area by muscle needling techniques.

Once abdominal muscle tension presents, tension needling is applied on the cross line on the abdominal muscles. Finding the tension line is very important to this technique. After loosening the abdominal muscle crossing point, the practitioner will press down on the legs in order to adjust the skin level. If a patient has leg problems, the practitioner will align the midline, treat the lengthened muscle line, and loosen the tight muscle and skin.

GIR treatment is used as the essential therapy in type M2 for restoring the breathing muscles. This method is explained in detail elsewhere. A certain amount of light pressure and slight sliding motions according to the patient's breathing can help to relax the tension of the abdominal and thoracic areas.

Type M2 is linked to internal conditions, especially internal pressure such as bloating, ascites, pregnancy, or indigestion. If the condition involves the digestive system, I sometimes ask patients to skip meals until the stomach gurgles. Acute, side-radiating back muscle pain is often caused by intestinal problems; prior referred pain should be ruled out to prevent further medical complications.

Simple Home Care and Cautions

Type M2 patients are recommended to passively stretch by using a pillow. Passive stretching is aided by gravity, with a partner or mechanical devices. While lying down on your side, place a pillow under your side chest area and wait one to two minutes. Raise your arm, move it forward and backward, and wave slowly. If tension is felt in a certain area while in a specific position, hold that position and breathe deeply. The intention is to make a smooth line on each section, such as from the armpit to the hip bone along the side line, from the collarbone to the lower abdomen along the front line, and from the neck to hip along the back line.

Change to the other side and adjust the level of the pillow to lower your waistline. Once you have completed both the right and left sides, move to your back and abdomen, following the same steps. Always remember the three dimensions of the body: side,

front, and back. You can even complete the steps while in a standing or sitting position by raising your arms over your head frequently.

Since type M2 patients have circular imbalances, especially in the torso area, focus your body's flexibility in all directions, not just in lengthening and strengthening. Try to balance your torso's outer shell first, and then your extremities. Leg exercise should be delayed until the sectional balance of your torso is achieved, as you can hurt your feet or knees due to misaligned muscles. It is preferable to get advice from a professional physical trainer if you wish to exercise.

Type M2 covers almost the entire outer shell of the body, so monitoring your skin's condition is recommended. Touch your skin daily and check the skin temperature with your hand, feel the texture, and take note of the blood vessel flow, color, and wrinkles.

You may find that one area of your knee is cooler than the other. For example, you may find a temperature difference between the front, back, and side. When you do find a colder area, simply rub it with your hands and hold for 30 seconds. Feet, ankles, knees, sides of legs, lower back, and side of the back are usual cold spots.

As previously discussed, type M2 is affected by the digestive system. If you are anxious or you find that you become anxious easily, your upper middle abdominal area may have congestion. It is advised that you reduce meal portion sizes, and warm up your upper abdomen by slightly pressing it and sliding downwards. If you suffer from depression, you can try standing up, raising your arms, and standing on your tiptoes. Relax and repeat this motion several times, or simply walk empty-handed, without bags, and try not to pick up your children or take your dog for a walk, for a while. A feeling of depression is often associated with an empty feeling caused by insufficient venous return, due to a sedentary or static sitting posture. By raising your arm, you can aid your breathing, and by standing on your tiptoes and relaxing, you can help circulate blood toward your heart.

With regard to type M2, many different etiologies can possibly be involved with symptoms and signs, and a serious problem is clearly exposed. If you have multiple symptoms and signs associated with type M2, you are in need of medical care or counseling.

Case Study

This case study involves a 44-year-old female.

Brief History

The patient reported that she experienced severe pain in her right shoulder 10 years earlier, but x-ray showed that the structure was normal. A doctor diagnosed it as myofascial pain and prescribed painkillers and recommended alternative therapies. The patient underwent 10 sessions of chiropractic therapy and 20 sessions of Chinese tuina massage therapy. Therapies were beneficial.

The pain had been lingering but did not interfere with her daily life.

Back and shoulder pain reappeared once she began a new job and worsened when she stood or used her hands for extended periods. She tried trigger-point therapy with another practitioner for several months. It dramatically changed her condition. After two to three days of treatment, the pain subsided almost completely. The effects of the treatment helped her to continue in her new job.

As her schedule was very busy, she was not able to commit to regular treatments, and only went for treatment whenever the symptoms reappeared. The duration of pain relief seemed to become shorter as she progressed with the treatment. Her back pain was not as severe as her shoulder pain. Eventually, a large circular mass was found in her shoulder. A friend recommended an alternative treatment, body shape change treatment, and thought it would help reduce the chronic pain, and so she came to see me.

She had a history of a C-section; the scar is horizontal across her lower abdomen. Other than that, she felt that she was healthy. She had a healthy family history. Both parents enjoyed their lifestyle with no need for medical care.

Observations

The first impression of her was narrow shoulders with a protruding chest and abdomen. Her posture was not bad, but her arm motion was somewhat narrow in range. Her complexion was pale with dark circles under her eyes. Her hair and skin appeared dry. She pointed out the area of shoulder pain on her right side. A mass the size of a ping-pong ball could be palpated. During palpation, she did not complain of any pain or pressure. Her range of motion and right side shoulder abduction seemed a little abnormal when she attempted to raise her arm and neck muscles simultaneously.

She had a scar on her lower abdomen that was a prominently fatty shape. The tube shape of the fat deposit ran across her entire waistline. The area between her rib cage and pelvis seemed to be all connected, and limited range was displayed when bending sideways and twisting her torso.

When she lay down on her abdomen, her sacral bone and hip areas were prominent and the upper thoracic area (T2–T9) was very tight and discolored. Right and left rear sides of armpits had tense skin, fatty tissue, and lymphatic water congestion. There were two active wrinkles and some inactive wrinkles. Her triceps were lengthened and her skin was less flexible on the left side. Her legs were swollen but not pitted. The areas behind her knees were especially tight. Her body shape presented with a small torso and long legs.

Assessment and Plan

Her shoulder pain was due to back pain. When examining her lower back, while she lay on her abdomen, it was hard to distinguish her waist and hip line, but it was visible when she lay on her back. Her lower back displayed several dark lines with wrinkles and connected toward the side of the body that had various conditions. The side with stretch marks and local congestion extended toward the lower abdominal fat. The quality of fat and congestion differed.

In a supine position, her abdomen had tension and her lower rib cage protruded. She had acne on her chest. Her body was types M2 and P, because her internal abdominal tension affected her rib cage and pelvis. Since her hands and arms were not involved in the posture and she did not have deep wrinkles on her neck, her shoulder pain may have resulted from the rotating arm movement.

I started treating her abdominal area with GIR to loosen tension first, and needled the rear side of her armpit wrinkles. Many responses occurred. The side tension congestion was treated with subcutaneous needling

and scraping to generate heat. I needled on her lower abdomen to loosen the abdominal muscle cross points. I then observed her legs, ankles, and feet. She had straight legs and I did not find any points of concern. If she had had any problems, I would have focused treatment on her ASIS area.

After several GIR treatments, her three muscle meridian lines were adjusted and moxa oil scraping was performed on her skin in order to loosen tightened areas. Her case was not severe and she has managed her health well. Sudden stress and overeating resulted in abdominal bloating and tension, and internal tension affected the structure of her body's outer shell. Because the torso is flexible, it is able to be re-formed.

TYPE M3 (FIGURE 6.7)

Quick Tips

1. When lying down and relaxed on your bed, try to wiggle your toes smoothly and gently spread them apart without involving your ankles and knees. If you have difficulty with gentle movement and struggle to move quickly, then you fall into type M3.
2. Again, in a lying-down position, relax your entire body and try to move your ankles very slowly in all directions, in a 360° circular motion. If this motion is difficult for you, you can be classified as type M3.
3. Bend your ankles toward your legs and stretch them. You may experience areas of tightness on your legs.
4. Check the bottoms and sides of your feet between your toes; are there any points of concern?

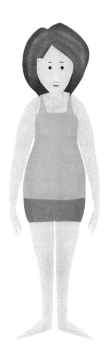

FIGURE 6.7
Type M3.

Related Condition

- Weakened pelvic floor: After childbirth, incorrect exercise, trauma
- Overactive bladder syndrome
- Constipation: Idiopathic or sphincter contraction
- Inner knee pain and swelling
- Whole-body pain: Fibromyalgia
- Lower back pain
- Heel and toe pain
- Occiput headache
- Gynecological issues, male fertility issues
- Lower abdominal scar from surgery
- Surgery on lower extremities and spent much time recovering
- Tightened gluteus muscles and leg muscles
- Swollen legs, especially inner thigh
- Balance problem
- Lower body obesity
- Swollen legs due to an internal organ disorder

Clinical Syndrome

Most type M3 syndromes demonstrate abnormal conditions on the lower extremities, such as swelling or local obesity, muscle tightness, and foot and toe problems. Patients may visit clinics in order to treat various symptoms, such as knee pain, hip pain, sprained ankle, foot pain, lower abdominal cramps, frequent urination, idiopathic constipation, and weight loss.

Even with different symptoms and signs, I found similar patterns during observation and palpation. On the contrary, sometimes the knee pain or leg pain is the same in terms of symptom, but the etiologies or body structures differ from each other. For example, both type M2 and type M3 exhibit

5. Have you recently experienced any pain, stiffness, or numbness in your big toe, without any other medical issues, such as diabetes? Does one or both of your feet have a bunion, a bump on the side of the big toe? It will appear as your big toe leans in toward the second toe, rather than pointing straight ahead.
6. Do you have heel pain accompanied by spider veins and a tendency to easily bruise on your legs? Palpate each side of your ankle; if your inner ankle feels swollen, follow along the tibia with light pressure. Do you feel pain or discomfort? Are your veins prominent? If you have a leg massage, you will probably feel tightness and tension.
7. Does your job consist of standing for long periods, or do you walk on a hard floor such as marble, tile, and stone throughout the day?

leg and foot discomfort and signs distinguishing the patterns. However, if the entire body structure is observed, we can find differences in character.

The leg structure of type M3 is different from that of type M2, which is closer to a valgus type. The key distinction is that a knock-knee can absorb the shock and flat feet can avoid further movement for type M2. Type M3's leg structure shows the opposite conditions. First, leg muscles are lengthened and weak, especially the gastrocnemius and soleus (back side of muscle connected with the Achilles tendon) muscles, and feel shrunken when palpated. The side and front leg muscles—the tibialis anterior, extensor digitorum longus, and extensor hallucis longus (extension for toes)—are lengthened and difficult to distinguish, which means the toes are misaligned and have limited motion. This causes the outside leg to tighten, and development of a hyperextended knee causes the patient to stand on the outside of the foot.

Usually the joint takes on the role as a shock absorber while we are in motion. If the knee is hyperextended and ankle inversion is present, which is caused by the foot supination in type M3, then each motional shock goes directly to the pelvic area and spine.

Clinical experience tells us that these conditions result from the tightness of hip muscles and the lower back pressing forward, which sets the hips and spine out of alignment. Comparing type M2 and type M3 lordosis cases, the lower back of type M3 patients does not necessarily present as an anterior pelvic tilt, which reduces the shock directly exerted on the spine. The anterior pelvic tilt is the body's natural way of maintaining flexibility, protecting the spine, and making more room for tension absorption, as in lordosis during pregnancy.

Instead of lordosis symptoms, kyphosis (hunched upper back) and scoliosis (sideways curvature of spine) are accompanied by type M3 disorders. In severe cases, a flat-back posture can be presented in conjunction with other symptoms. A typical flat-back posture is a forward-leaning head, long neck shape (cervical spine extended), straight chest and back, posterior tilted pelvis, extended hip and knees, and ankle joint inversion.

The appearance of someone in a flat-back posture is sometimes also apparent. It is rather common in people who tend to perform many sit-up-type exercises, boxers, and those who have poor core and back stability. They tend to be very alert and have quick responses and high endurance. Most patients incline more to the fight and flight mode, rather than the relax and rest mode.

The type M3 group has internal symptoms related to gynecologic issues, urinary and bowel syndromes, and circulatory problems, such as insufficiency of venous return. Unlike other groups, type M3 patients do not complain of pain in its initial stage; however, over an extended period, the pain may become intense and unbearable.

It is important to record the medical history, which may consist of trauma, injury, or any surgery, to assess the treatment plan for type M3. Type M3 symptoms are presented on the entire body if in the chronic stage, and outer appearances are not as prominent as they are in types M1 and M2.

Lower extremities support your balance, side by side, front, and back, constantly moving and adjusting motion to maintain the correct position for your upper body. These endeavors are influenced by any biomechanical changes or stresses on the pelvic region, which is the center of information between the legs and spine. Feet, ankles, knees, lower abdominal area, groin area, and thoracic and lumbar spine problems can lead to movement compensations, which can change the normal function of the pelvis and legs. Over time, these changes result in abnormal hip joint structures.

Type M3 displays conditions similar to those of a pear-shaped body. The hip and pelvic upper thigh areas look larger than other parts of the body. Especially, the area between the legs bulges with extra fatty tissue and cellulite. If the congestion or obesity symptoms are severe, the outer shape is similar to that of an anterior pelvic tilt, X-shaped legs, and even a flat-footed shape. However, if you palpate the legs and pelvis area, the internal muscles and vein conditions will exhibit symptoms associated with type M3. Types S, M2, and M3 can present simultaneously, and so do their symptoms. In such cases, the treatment will be processed externally from the outer shell and move inward, toward the internal organs.

Understanding the Mechanism

Type M3 is related to the vertically aligned pathway along the feet to the cervical spine, following the circulatory system (Figure 6.8). Whereas type M1 involves the horizontal arm and shoulder rotation, leading the breathing muscles, type M2 lengthens and is strengthened with a circular accordion-shaped cylinder in the outer shell of the body.

The pelvis is the center of the body, linking the spine and the legs. The information received from the bottom of the body is gathered at the pelvis and transferred to the brain. Orders are received from the brain at the pelvis and are enacted by the lower extremities. If the pelvis is weak and has a problem, the entire body can be affected.

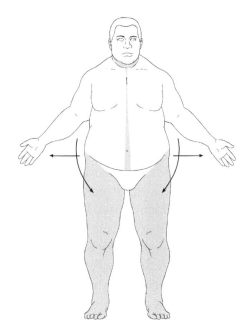

FIGURE 6.8
Type M3 mechanism.

For example, a misplaced and weak pelvic diaphragm results in pain and tension, which will affect breathing and freedom of movement.

Body Balance

During an ordinary stance, the pelvis is tipped slightly forward, controls the whole-body equilibrium, and maintains an upright posture. When the balance is disturbed by either an external or internal force, the body immediately reacts in order to move the trunk and extremities and so find a stable center. A stable center is changeable, depending on the motion and action.

Balancing, in essence, means the constant communication of each side and the negotiating of the center of power between the two sides. The body has three major control mechanisms for body balance and posture: one is control over the whole-body equilibrium to maintain an upright posture, another is control over lumbopelvic orientation to maintain spinal posture, and the last is control at the intervertebral level to maintain vertebral body alignment.

When picking up a heavy object from the ground with your arms, the internal force between the trunk and lower extremities is reactive. If a bus or train stops suddenly, your extremities will grab a secure object or readjust your standing position in order to resist the forward moving force and so regain balance. Since every movement demands control of equilibrium, trunk and spinal flexibility and stability are necessary. The center base for the two vertical equilibrium lines (one on the right side of the leg toward the spine, the other on the left side of the leg toward the spine) is the pelvis.

Muscle Sequential Connection and Function for Type M3

The erector spinae muscle provides resistance and assists in the control of bending forward at the waist level. As it is named, an erect position from bending is carried out by the erector spinae extensors. The erector spinae muscle consists of three columns of muscle, the iliocostalis, longissimus, and spinalis, each running parallel on the outer sides of the vertebra and extending from the lower back of the skull all the way down to the pelvis.

The erector spinae muscle has many antagonist and synergist muscle groups as the muscles cover almost the entire back area, connecting the neck, ribs, and pelvis. The antagonists at the neck are the neck flexors, such as the sternocleidomastoid, the longus coli, and the longus capitis. The rectus abdominis and the abdominal oblique muscles are the antagonists for trunk action. While straightening the spine, the synergists are the hip extensors (gluteus maximus muscles) and the hamstring muscles. The erector spinae muscle triggers pain over your entire back and may even send pain to your upper leg and lower abdominal region.

The hamstrings are located on the back of the thighs. They are composed of three muscles. On the inside of the thighs are the semimembranosus and semitendinosus. On the outside are the biceps femoris. The hamstrings originate from the lower pelvic bone, and they connect with the pelvis, the femur, and the lower leg. If you bend your knee into a sitting position, the hamstring contracts.

When you sit on a chair, you can move your ankle in a motion similar to that of pressing the brake pedal in your car. Your back leg muscles engage in this motion. The back leg muscles are the gastrocnemius and soleus muscles. Both the gastrocnemius and the soleus run the entire length of the lower leg, connecting behind the knee and at the heel.

The gastrocnemius muscles have two branches at the top behind the knee and connect medially and laterally with the thighbone, the femur. During walking, the gastrocnemius muscle is flexed and creates the bending action for smooth movement of the upper legs. If you wear high heels or flip-flops, the knee bending motion will be decreased.

Both the gastrocnemius muscle and the soleus join onto the Achilles tendon, which is one of most important parts for balancing in an upright posture. The ankle, the approximately six-inch circular lower leg compartment, can affect your static body posture, motion, walking, and balancing because the area includes almost 10 tendons, many ligaments, nerves, and blood vessels communicating with the central nervous system through the vibration of tendons, venous return, and skeletomuscular imbalance.

In TCM and Asian culture, the feet and lower legs have been treated as the symbol of a healthy life and longevity. If you keep your feet warm and clean, your important tendons will not become stiff and rigid, and blood circulation will be encouraged.

Type M3 focuses on the lower extremity–pelvis–spine loop mechanisms. The causative factors that occur at the root of the loop can result in symptoms. For example, an individual had to have knee surgery due to an accident, and one leg became weaker than the other because of a long recovery period. The individual only used one leg, and as a result, the body compensated for this irregularity. The lumbar muscles became contracted in the inactive leg. This caused postural problems with a poor walking gait. The poor walking gait generated leg joint pain and foot pain that was felt in the spine.

As another example, a patient had a myomectomy for uterine fibroids several years ago and subsequently had another surgery for endometriosis. Since then, she felt skin tightness on the one side, mostly due to scarring on the skin area, and she tried to avoid bending the area, so she stretched her spine as much as possible. Later, she had severe pain in the occipital area and ankle, which continued until her lower pelvic area was treated.

Type M3 and Blood Circulation

An important characteristic in type M3 is the relationship between the muscles and the blood vessel pump. The legs have several skeletal pumps for circulation to assist the venous return, which is toward the right atrium after pushing venous blood up with muscular contraction. If there is limited muscle contraction in the lower extremities, blood can pool in the lower legs. This causes a decrease in the venous return and cardiac output.

Especially ankle movements such as plantar flexion and dorsi flexion (heel and toe position) are triggers to move the gastrocnemius muscle, passing the central vein between the two areas of the muscle. But a poor range of motion in an ankle occurs in conditions where muscles are already lengthened or weakened, by wearing uncomfortable shoes such as high heels, and swollen ankles. Furthermore, long periods of standing and sitting may also result in insufficient venous return.

A chronic insufficient venous return results in edema, swelling, and skin changes. In this case, one-third of the lower leg may display spider veins, discoloration, ulcers, and thinning skin. Toe movement will be limited, and sometimes the toe shape is deformed.

Ankle and toe movement are closely related because the muscles of toe extensors work together when the ankle is extended and the muscles of the toe flexors work with the ankle flexors. However, the toe extensor and flexor muscles move freely while the ankle muscles rest.

This means that if the ankle muscles do not have a full range of motion, toe motions are restricted. Toe pain or deformity influences the position of the ankles and knees, which will affect the walking gait and the entire body.

One-third of leg components are mostly tendons, which tend to be poor blood supply areas. A lack of blood supply will not allow rapid eradication of swollen symptoms. The daily care of ankles and feet is the best way to prevent type M3 symptoms.

Pain

Type M3 patients do not usually complain of pain symptoms during the initial stages. When they do notice the pain, the incident that led to the problem is usually long forgotten if not related to an accident or trauma. The pain is not localized, and it is easy to pinpoint the origin. It does not involve inflammation or muscle contractions.

Type M3 patients usually experience pain in the occiput area and complain of shoulder pain, upper back pain, lower back pain, pelvic pain, leg pain, medial and lateral knee pain, and ankle pain. Their pain is quite intense and affects their daily life. Sometimes spastic pain and muscle spasms bother them at night and cause sleep interference, which can cause depression.

Type M3 pain characteristics are as follows: Before the pain began, patients were very active, athletic, and maintained a busy schedule, enjoying sports and dancing. Mild discomforts such as constipation, foot pain, and shoulder pain did not bother their activities. The common pain trigger is time off from daily activities. For example, a sprained ankle may have triggered entire body pain after spending several days off. Or a stressful project was completed and time was taken off for a vacation. Or emotional trauma caused by a breakup or separation resulted in physical pain after suffering the emotional pain. While going through a difficult time, type M3 patients typically lose weight and severe pain begins.

In my clinical experience, the physical patterns are found and the pain spot is usually showed by stretched muscle fibers and a "dried-out" body fluids area. This is not treated with trigger point needling. The muscles alongside the spine are very tight and the spine cannot move freely. At the same time, the inner legs and thigh areas are very sensitive to pressure. When areas of pain are stimulated or palpated, the real pain spot will react.

For example, one of my patients complained of upper neck pain, but her neck and arms did not have any points of concern. While I palpated her neck, the left side of her hip muscles twitched. I went on to record her history and understand her condition. She had been severely traumatized by second surgery complications, and 15 years previously, she suffered several pelvic organ issues. She had been so busy taking care of children that she did not have much time to focus on her own health care. The pelvic pain affected her walking and standing posture. Her spine transformed to a flat-back shape. She had chronic indigestion and constipation. She reported never feeling real relaxation.

The root cause of the pain that she experienced was chronic sacral tension stress from lower extremity movement. Her lower abdominal tension and discomfort were related to the lower back as it stretched and minimized the impact on the abdominal scarring area. This brought about the discomfort and pain sensation. By aligning her leg muscles, loosening the hip muscles, relaxing her skin and spine, and employing scar treatment, I was able to reduce her symptoms.

The case is related to adhesion-related disorder, which is a complex of symptoms related to adhesions. It is usually discovered when the patient's primary complaint is chronic abdominal pain. Their symptoms can be primarily in one area of the abdomen, but are often generalized, vague cramps and difficult to define. Sometimes other intestinal problems accompany the pain.

Type M3 patients can rarely indicate the exact location of the pain, but the area of pain can be easily palpated on the inner ankle, inner legs and knees, hip muscles, iliotibial (IT) band, lower abdomen, and upper neck. Hip pain tends to be in the medial area and anterior of the hip. Posterior and lateral pain is often referred from the lumbar spine or sacroiliac joints.

Type M3 pain is not easy to treat once it is exhibited. Prevention is of utmost importance.

Postural Characteristics

- Face: Double chin, tight closed mouth, and staring eyes
- Neck: Front part of neck has wrinkles (many lines), erect neck posture, long neck
- Arms: Weak muscle tone
- Hands and fingers: Weak muscle tone
- Skin: Overall dark complexion, easily bruised, purple or blue color of skin near the veins of the lower extremities
- Blood vessel: Expanded inner leg and ankle blood vessel varicose veins
- Range of motion: Toe and ankle movement is not smooth, knee hyperextended or knee extended outer, limited hip flexion
- Spine: Scoliosis, kyphosis, overall spinal tension, stretched spine
- Behavior: Quick reactions
- Fat distribution: Upper hip (differs from lower back area), inner legs, lower abdomen, urogenital area, and thigh

Possible Associated Disorders

- Fibromyalgia
- Idiopathic dizziness
- Pelvic floor disorder
- Pelvic congestion syndrome
- Phleboliths in the pelvis
- Bunions
- Insufficient venous return syndrome
- Scoliosis and kyphosis
- Hip strain
- Adhesion-related disorders

Treatment

The three foot yin muscle tendon meridians are used in diagnosis and as a treatment guideline for type M3 syndrome. The three foot yin meridians begin at the soles of the feet and follow along the inner leg and thigh and the front part of the ASIS and cover the urogenital area in the pelvic cavity and the midline of the lower abdomen. They connect with the inner spinal ligament and bind at the occipital bone. Most meridian paths will be observed and palpated before and during the treatment period.

The aims of treatment for type M3 are

1. Find the hidden pain and the origin of the loop.
2. Relax hypertonia.
3. Restore flexibility.
4. Improve circulation.
5. Harmonize body balance.
6. Increase strength.

A health history and current body expression are important clues in finding the loop connection that is repeated as a vicious cycle, the cause to result to the result to cause. The older and newly developed symptomatic issues tend to be treated at the same time. If the old problem is abdominal pain and the current issue is neck pain, the abdomen and neck should be treated at the same time during each session.

The type M3 mechanism is the foot to upper neck area, the vertical and internal balance system. For this reason, the hypertonic area is present if the body has been out of balance. The usual spot for the hypertonic area is around the joint area, which may result in abnormal swelling and muscle development.

Since the spine is involved in upright postural balance, Du meridian (channel flow on spine) and erector spinae muscles may be directly treated with the muscle meridian needling technique, and other modalities will be applied to the spine.

For balancing treatment, loosening of the pelvic area is paramount and the treatment will be spread out upward and downward, especially gathering and narrowing at the "bottleneck" spot, which is indicated as several tendons and muscles crossing or passing closely, such as in the inner knee area (hamstring and gastrocnemius muscles). Muscle and tendon lining alignment treatment will be applied if the line is misaligned.

For relaxing the physical tension, GIR treatment is followed by any appropriate treatment modality in each session. If scar tissue is present, scar tissue treatment will also be applied.

For patient home care, postural corrections will be taught in a standing and a lying-down position.

Simple Home Therapy and Precautions

For type M3 patients, nightly feet and ankle care is recommended. Clean and scrub the toes, between the toes, the soles of the feet, the sides of the feet, the ankles, and the legs with a small rough towel or brush. Then dry the skin and check the flexibility of your feet, ankles, and knees. Sleep with socks on.

Whenever in a lying-down position, relax your entire body and focus only on your toes. Start to wiggle your toes like a butterfly; very gently and smoothly move them without moving your ankles. The knees and ankles should also be relaxed. Even if your movements are small, they will be beneficial. Just relax and wiggle your toes for two minutes. Then you can begin to move your ankles in a circular motion, very gently and slowly for three minutes. After treatment, the pelvis and legs will begin to loosen. This home care will be recommended by the practitioner.

For ballet posture number 1, the heels touch each other and the feet face outward, as though trying to form a straight line. Your feet should be turned outward only as far as they are comfortable, and the soles of your feet and your toes should be in contact with the floor. Once you are in ballet posture number 1, contract your anus tightly. Then stretch your spine and point your chin upward. That is the initial stage of vertical stretching for type M3 syndrome.

Once type M3 upright posture is comfortable, followed motions are added for entire body balance.

1. Type M3: Assume ballet posture number 1.
2. Type M2: Lengthen or stretch abdominal circular cylinder.
3. Type M1: Open palms of your hands and rotate your palms outward.

Patients are asked to perform and practice these sequential motions at home. It is important to perform these motions after treatment.

Case Study

This case study involves a 33-year-old female.

Observations

On her first visit, February 8, 2012, the patient complained of lower back pain and heartburn since her mid-20s. Menstrual cramps and pain were aggravated during menstruation. She reported that lower back pain was understandable, but heartburn was not acceptable. A gastrointestinal checkup had not found any problems, but whenever heartburn occurred, she took over-the-counter (OTC) medication. She had been taking a birth control pill for about 12 years and allergy medication when experiencing hay fever. She drank wine occasionally, perhaps once a week.

She is a designer, uses a computer, and sits for long periods, as she prefers to complete a project without distractions. She played basketball and volleyball in high school and college. She enjoys activities but does not have much opportunity to engage in them because she works during the day and teaches classes to students two nights a week. Her eating habits are regular and include healthy foods. She believes she is healthy, except for the heartburn and lower back pain.

She had her spine x-rayed and has visited other medical practitioners. She did not get much information regarding the pain in relation to her bone structure and discomfort. The x-ray showed no problems with her spine. Furthermore, the patient mentioned that she always felt cold. She wore a long shirt, cardigan, long pants, and two pairs of socks, boots, and a scarf.

Regarding her medical history, during childhood, she had sudden leg muscle weakness and could not walk straight. She remembered that she had a brace on her right leg for several months.

She suffered from a plant allergy.

The patient came across as analytical, had a strong mental ego, and displayed a well-planned attitude toward her lifestyle. She worked for a stable company and received a good salary. She was financially and socially well off. Overall, she was satisfied with her lifestyle and believed herself capable of doing as she wished. She felt that if there was any way to resolve her chronic discomfort, she would endeavor to do just that.

Brief History

My first impression of her was that she was tall and slim, except in her hip area. She had a long neck, but a V-shaped clavicle. Her skin color was pale with no wrinkles. She was referred by another patient who had gastrointestinal problems, and she indicated that she wanted to resolve her stomach bloating and the discomfort of the heartburn she was experiencing.

While palpating and manipulating her abdomen, I felt only thick mass, like tensed skin. I could not reach any other muscles. The surface of her skin was very smooth but extremely tense; I had never encountered such tension. She was very proud of the condition of her skin, and she said that she applied lotion daily. However, I found a vast difference in the condition of the skin on her lower back and down toward her legs. These areas had many stretch marks and pores. Stretch marks were present from the iliac crest area and down toward the back of her thigh on both sides of her body. Her pelvic and thigh area were larger than her torso, but she was very slim from the knees downward, similar to her arms.

Her neck was straight and her lower back had the appearance of lumbar lordosis, but the skin congestion and tightness prevented palpation. Her spinal gap was narrow and her spinal muscles were very tight, even though she had excess subcutaneous fat on her back.

Unlike the previous medical diagnosis of her spine, the patient's movement was an important clue in treatment. Her upper body (torso) was locked while she walked. Type M3 patients usually experience a lack of movement and flexibility that extends from the upper thoracic region to the cervical area. Their posture and walking gait often resemble those of a military soldier. Type M3 female patients frequently express satisfaction with their upper bodies because they have a long neck and their torsos are not larger than their lower bodies. However, these female patients will often wish to alter their appearance by getting rid of their "fat hip or thigh areas." The patient mentioned had she had tried to get rid of her cellulite with exercise, but failed attempts caused her to give up.

Although type M3 features were more prominent, she also had type T and P signs and symptoms. I explained to her that her condition was similar to that of a balloon filled with too much air and would possibly burst due to the excess pressure.

Even though she had an even skin tone and complexion between her breast and umbilicus area, she did exhibit two dark wrinkles that run horizontally. These lines were faint on the side of her body. Her upper chest and abdomen area were thinner than the lower half of her body, which was a cylinder shape. While lying down, her abdomen and rib cage movement were rather weak, and no breathing muscle action was visible. Her eyes were wide open, and she constantly talked and asked questions. At first, I just thought she was nervous about her environment and the treatment. However, after a year, this behavior was still very apparent.

I noticed that when she lay on her back, she was not entirely comfortable; there was a large gap between her waist and the bed. It was as if she was lying on an imaginary pillow. She previously mentioned that her spine and back appeared to be perfectly fine. I noticed that a long and deep skinfold had developed. The imaginary pillow effect that I mentioned earlier is caused by the adipose tissue connected to the latissimus dorsi muscle and gluteus maximus muscle, causing chronic water accumulation and stretching the skin in several horizontal directions. I did not count exactly how many lines were present, but there appeared to be more than 15.

Interestingly, her thoracolumbar fascia, which is on the mid–lower back area, was not affected by the so-called pillow. More "pillows" were found on the medial and lateral side of her thigh and between the humerus and scapula, mostly on the rotator cuff muscles. She displayed a normal range of motion in all directions. However, while in the supine posture, she had difficulty moving her hands and arms.

Assessment and Treatment

Her neck and hip state clearly indicated type M3, as her neck was straightened and lengthened, the gluteus muscles were stretched, and a depression between the inguinal region and tensor fascia latae was visible. In comparing the shoulder and hip circumference, the shoulder and upper thoracic area were tight and small, whereas the hip region was larger.

On the medial side of her thigh, fatty tissue accumulation indicated that her pelvic diaphragm was stretched and her hamstring was lengthened and possibly attached to the gracilis muscle or other adhesions. Once these areas were loosened, a practitioner would be able to easily gain access to the muscles and the problem area in order to effectively palpate them.

Her chronic physical stress made her easily anxious, and this frustrated her. Her emotional tension was as severe as were her skin manifestation. Type P displays more tension of the body and emotions, more so than any other types. Type P has several different shapes; her case included "tension on torso and loosened on extremities." There were also some allergic reactions and heartburn that were closer to type T. I began to treat her based on my assessment centered on the six body types. My conclusion was types M3 and P.

If type M and other physiologic symptoms of types P, T, and S are combined, the priority is the latter, because anatomical structure corrections follow the internal organ condition.

For type P, loosening tension in the torso and extremities, usually abdominal and pelvic cavities, is the first target. Patients are easily annoyed with any stimulation and pain tolerance is very low.

I treated her abdomen first. GIR was used in three sessions. Then she started to listen to my instruction and her condition improved. I added hyperthermal therapy with GIR to induce sweating. An infrared dome was used with a blanket that covered only her abdominal area, because her rib cage and diaphragm were not fully functioning for breathing and transferring lymphatic fluids.

After hyperthermal therapy, her abdominal pressure eased. Once the symptoms of type P were improving, she mentioned that she wanted to stop the birth control pill. She tried to eliminate alcohol and heed sleep time regulation. She even took regular baths at home. Her attitude was very different from the day we first met. She started walking many miles in San Francisco downtown. Whenever she walked a great distance, she had leg pain; the pain scale was usually 5/10, and the quality was shooting local pain and achy on the side of her legs and spread outward. Her knee was overextended and locked. When she had been walking and bathing for several months, she still felt cold and did not sweat much. Her skin had not changed much.

As soon as she started exercise and a half-body bath, her allergy symptoms flared up severely. The allergy symptoms included a runny nose, itchy eyes, and sore throat triggered by cold weather and plants, she insisted, because she had an allergy test in the hospital. Even her back pain was worse. After she suffered severe allergic symptoms, she met her ob-gyn to change her birth control mode.

Her waistline was smaller than before treating type M3. Digestion issues had been alleviated.

In October 2014, I started to treat her type M3 symptoms. The type M3 treatment combined two modalities. One was moxa oil cream scraping gua sha, and the other cupping and muscle meridian needling. Following the three foot yin meridian, I scraped with moxa oil and needled between the anterior superior iliac spine and the femur lateral trochanter. Once gua sha and needling are done, the patient needs to stand in ballet pose number 1, which is feet turned out only as far as is comfortable and the sole of the foot and toes in contact with the floor.

Her condition improved and she reported feeling much warmer and being able to wear a sleeveless shirt. Her back cushion, "the imaginary pillow," is gone and her rib cage moves while she breathes. She can control her schedule and tries to move as much as she can. Her body looks smoother and slimmer than before, and her upper and lower body are balanced.

7

Muscle Meridian Therapy and Skin Cutaneous Therapy

WHAT ARE MUSCLE AND SINEW MERIDIANS AND CUTANEOUS MERIDIANS?

As mentioned in Chapter 2, there are six meridian classifications based on similar tissue structures and functions. Before focusing on the meridian theories, we need to understand the tissues of the human body. Tissues are complex organisms and provide numerous functions necessary for organs to maintain life. Each tissue performs at least one unique function that helps maintain homeostasis. The body is formed with a "matrix of tissues" surrounded by or embedded in complex extracellular material. Our body wears several matrix garments that can consciously support survival and maintain life.

There are four major basic tissues in our body: epithelium, connective, muscular, and nervous.

1. **Epithelial tissue** forms the coverings of surfaces and lines body cavities. As such, it serves many purposes, including protection, absorption, excretion, secretion, filtration, and sensory reception.
2. **Muscle tissue** produces movement and is adapted for contractility and movement by shortening and lengthening.
3. **Nervous tissue** communicates between the various parts of the body and in integration of their activities.
4. **Connective tissue** is the most abundant and widely distributed tissue type found in the human body. It supports the body and its parts, connecting and holding them together. The role of connective tissue is to transport substances through the body, and to protect it from foreign invaders.

Classification of Connective Tissues

Connective tissue is one of the most widespread and diverse tissues in the body and is found in or around every organ of the body. It connects tissues to each other, muscles to muscles, muscles to bones, and bones to bones. One type of connective tissue, blood, transports nutrients to cells. Several other types of connective tissue cells defend against microorganisms and other invaders.

Connective tissues have been classified by histologists in several different ways:

1. Fibrous (connective tissue proper) includes loose connective tissue, adipose tissue, and reticular and dense connective tissue, such as collagen and elastin. In relation to this category are fascia, fat deposits, and allergies.
2. Bone.
3. Cartilage.
4. Blood.

Tissues and body membranes are referred to as the fabric of the body and make up a large part of the body's integrated structures. An essential function of most tissues and membranes is the maintenance of relative constancy in the body: homeostasis.

Meridian Classifications

The goal of acupuncture and moxibustion treatment is known as balancing the yin and yang in the body, especially as followed in various meridian therapies. The meridians are formed within the body matrix, connecting and transmitting internally and externally to support body function and structure.

The meridians are classified by their similar functions and structures:

- 12 cutaneous (skin) meridians
- 12 tendinomuscular (muscle) meridians
- Luo-connecting meridians*
- 12 divergent meridians
- 12 primary meridians (Jing)*
- 8 extraordinary meridians

Except for the 8 extraordinary meridians, the other meridians are grouped according to the 12 primary meridian flows and their names.

Six Body Types and Muscle Meridians

Since all the meridians connect together and communicate with each other, I choose the 12 muscle meridians and 12 cutaneous meridians to form part of body-reshaping treatments. The structural appearance of the body is easily detected by the surface skin and is formed by musculoskeletal muscle conditions.

When I treat patients, I focus on the 12 muscle meridians even though the other meridians are also used, as the muscle meridians follow the 12 primary meridian pathways. This allows me to observe the entire body rather than just the symptoms or signs. This makes diagnosis easier and treatment more effective. When I observe and palpate in order to diagnose, I take note of not only the skin, but also the connective tissue and muscles beneath it. The acupuncture needles penetrate through the

---

* In Chinese, the word *meridian* is the *Jing Luo*; *Jing* is represented as a vertical pathway and *Luo* is the web or network branching out from the Jing. These Jing Luo meridians span across body tissue and influence bioactive functions, which are known as Qi, and blood circulation in meridians.

skin and into muscle, which also affects the surrounding tissue, skin, and muscles.

For these reasons, the muscle meridian needling technique is unique to other acupuncture treatment techniques. The aim of the acupuncture needle is to target the area between the skin and muscle, or within the muscle fiber itself. When performing a muscle meridian treatment, it is necessary for me to obtain a needling sensation. This is done by slightly moving the needle around once it has been placed into the skin. Once the needling sensation is achieved, the needle is quickly removed.

Muscle meridian (and sinew) therapy originates in traditional Chinese medicine (TCM) and relates to musculoskeletal pain and atrophy or other problems in muscles and tendons. Muscle meridian therapy is not only for musculoskeletal pain treatment, but also treats most muscle atrophy conditions, such as paralysis of muscle from stroke. This technique is used to restore the imbalanced phasic lengthening of the muscle group for body reshaping.

Chronic muscle imbalances may result in deformed body structure. For example, excessive hunching over may cause conditions associated with chest depression or suppression. These may cause breathing capacity problems. You may wish to correct your posture; however, the stretched and lengthened back muscle and shortened front muscle may not allow for adequate balance. Sometimes your balance can be corrected by stretching and exercising, but in many cases, it is very difficult, as the lengthened muscle fibers cannot be restored simply by exercising or stretching. For this reason, the muscle meridian needling technique is very useful, as it effectively restores both lengthened and contracted muscles.

Although the muscle meridians are not directly connected to any major organs, muscle meridian therapy has been effective in restoring muscle forms and balanced movement after organ or tissue disorders. A restored body posture may positively affect the corresponding organ systems.

All muscle meridians originate from the end of distal body parts, such as fingers and toes, which perform the detailed expression and micromovement in our daily life. If you have a problem in your wrist, such as carpal tunnel syndrome, the root will be in the exact problem point or in another area along the movement line of your arm. It is possibly caused somewhere along the hand yin muscle meridian. If this problem is caused by abnormal congestion in the armpit area, the skin will display symptoms such as raised pores, the muscle will appear thin and tight, and the area will exhibit fat congestion. The best course of treatment is to loosen the muscle, tighten the skin, and resolve the congestion. Physical therapy and exercise deal with active muscle movement, while massage therapy and other manual therapies assume passive movement. Muscle meridian therapy is a more passive approach in dealing with musculoskeletal issues.

MUSCLE MERIDIAN TREATMENTS FOR SIX BODY TYPE GROUPS

For diagnosing and treating the six body types, muscle meridians are classified in four groups: three foot yang muscle meridians, three foot yin muscle meridians, three hand yang muscle meridians, and three hand yin muscle meridians (Figure 7.1).

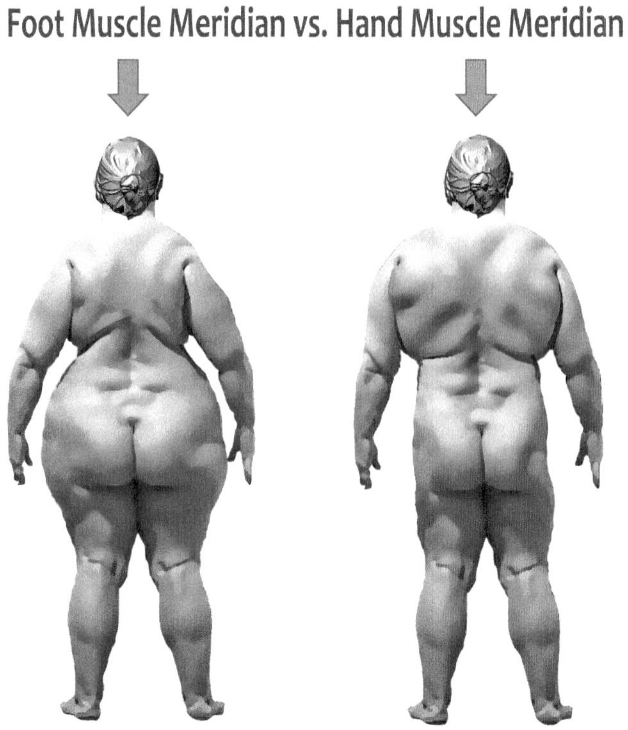

Foot Muscle Meridian vs. Hand Muscle Meridian

FIGURE 7.1
Muscle meridian pattern.

The three hand yang muscle meridians' pathogenic conditions are presented as muscle contraction and tightness of arms, upper shoulder, side of neck, and facial muscle. These meridians flow along the palms and inner arms toward the thoracic cavity and meet up in the diaphragm region. These muscle meridian pathogens are presented by armpit and upper chest congestion and circulation and breathing problems.

The three foot yang muscle meridians' pathogenic conditions originate from the abdominal area and on the same level of the side and back region. Lower back lordosis, fluid congestions with hidden stretch marks, and abdominal tension are common symptoms. These meridians flow from the soles of the feet to the heels and inner thighs, and pelvic and spinal regions. The pathogenic conditions contribute to foot pain, occiput head pain, or inner thigh weakness and pelvic muscle weakness. Inner thigh congestion or pelvic inflammation is sometimes also present.

Characteristics of Muscle Meridians

Nourish the Muscles, Tendons, and Skin

According to TCM books, muscle meridians nourish the muscles, tendons, and skin with Qi and blood. In other words, they do not indicate that muscle meridians make up the anatomical group of muscle or tendon, but the biomechanical and biophysical connections should be illustrated to better understand the systemic mechanisms. They communicate and have an effect on the skin and tendons to which the blood vessels are supplied and are protected by the muscles that flow parallel to the meridian.

In other words, the condition of the distal muscles, tendons, and skin can indicate the connective health between internal blood vessels and the nervous systems. Therefore, muscle meridian systems are useful for gathering information about systemic and holistic body mechanisms.

Three Yang and Three Yin Hand and Foot Meridians

Three yang and three yin meridians are present in each hand and foot and cover all the muscles and the entire surface of the body. The three yang hand muscle meridians are

- Hand Tai yang small intestine meridian
- Hand Shao yang triple burner meridian
- Hand Yang Ming large intestine meridian

The three yin hand muscle meridians are

- Hand Tai yin lung meridian
- Hand Shao yin heart meridian
- Hand Jue yin pericardium meridian

The three foot yang muscle meridians are

- Foot Tai yang urinary bladder meridian
- Foot Shao yang gallbladder meridian
- Foot Yang Ming stomach meridian

The three foot yin muscle meridians are

- Foot Tai yin spleen meridian
- Foot Shao yin kidney meridian
- Foot Jue yin liver meridian

All the muscle meridians flow similar to the main meridians. Muscle meridians and main meridians share a close relationship even though they are not connected to one another. Muscle meridians are the conduit to distribute the Qi and blood to the muscles, and they unite all the bones and joints of the body and maintain a normal range of motion.

Muscle Meridian Pathogenic Patterns

Although muscle meridians do not all correspond to anatomical muscle connections and fascia covers, they do explain the pathologic aspect of their structure and function in a practical way. It is more effective to explain it with regard to active motion and range of motion. Furthermore, when the muscle meridian is manifested, it is clear that a pathogenic condition is involved. For example, if two muscles are chronically weak and dystrophy is present, the gap between the two muscles will develop tension and soft tissue lines that can be observed in a clinic. A good example is the spot between the pectoralis major and deltoid anterior muscle. In a healthy condition, it is hard to find abnormal lines or spots.

Similar to all meridians, the disorder or pathologic condition can present an abnormal condition and a line may be formed. If you check your body thoroughly, you will see the difference between a normal and abnormal condition. Symptoms of restricted meridians are pulled, twisted, strained, and weak muscle; muscle dystrophy; muscle spasms; cramps; and the presence of a mass. Muscle meridians, according to the yin and yang theory, emphasize a balancing and interdependent function.

It has been stated in TCM literature that "when the yang is distressed, the yang meridian muscles become over extended, when yin is distressed, the yin meridian muscles are contracted." Furthermore, "when there is cold, the muscles become tense, when there is heat, muscles become lax." These two sentences are important clues in developing muscle meridian treatment plans in my clinic.

Observations of agonist and antagonist muscles and yin and yang muscle groups clearly illustrate pathologic symptoms, especially in those who have a poor posture or limited range of motion. For example, people who have gained weight and experienced a change in body shape will experience an extension in all foot and hand yang meridians and a contraction in all foot and hand yin meridians.

Muscle Meridians Originate from Distal Body Parts

Muscle meridians originate from the extremities of the limbs and ascend to the head and trunk. Unlike anatomical separation, large disperses to small. You need to think, "The little things make up the big thing." The small movements of the fingers and toes can cause large movements, according to the muscle meridian theory.

When you move your finger, tendons and muscles connected to your hand and forearm move even though other, larger muscle groups are relaxed. Moreover, if you start to move your wrist, then a larger muscle group is involved in the movement, yet your shoulder and upper arm muscles remain relaxed. Individual joint, tendon, and muscle movement is an important checkpoint; however, the muscle meridian is explained by more than the joint motions.

The distal part of the body has the directional characteristic function, which means your extremities are following the hand and feet leading the way. For example, when you turn your arm upside down, it will be hard to do so without your hand's cooperation. If you rotate your arm outwards or inwards, leading with your fingers and hand is relatively easier than trying to move your arm with your shoulder and upper arm while your hand remains static. The leading of the distal hand and foot can be decided to direct your entire extremity's action. Skeletal muscle functions form part of a well-organized society, free to embrace individualism and collaborate for the most economical way of achieving a common goal.

The distal body health condition can be determined by internal body organ conditions such as peripheral blood circulation or peripheral neuropathy. In this case, observing the entire muscle meridian flow is needed to treat the local congestion or systemic disorder.

On the contrary, the condition of the distal area can affect organ systems, such as venous return disorder. The flow of the muscle meridian is toward the torso, similar to the venous system and lymph system movement, and is followed by muscle working, such as the ankle and gastrocnemius venous pump action.

Muscle Meridian

Muscle meridian treatment is not for treating individual muscle contraction or muscle fibers; its purpose is to determine the condition of the entire muscle meridian group and observe and palpate the connection line. When dealing with a pathogenic condition in the meridians, you can observe or palpate the differences compared to normal conditions. Therefore, the diagnostic posture is very important when checking the muscle meridian conditions. I will briefly discuss the diagnosis posture in my clinical observation of each meridian.

Three Hand Yang Meridians

For six body types treatments, the three hand yang meridians are used in type M1 yang diagnosis, treatment, and prognosis.

- Clinical syndrome in three hand yang meridians
- Winged scapular
- Kyphosis
- Temporomandibular disorder (TMD)
- Hearing problem (earache)
- Chronic sinus congestion
- Upper body and shoulder pain

Hand Tai Yang Small Intestine Meridian Flow (Figure 7.2)

Pathway: Little finger → wrist → forearm → elbow → medial condyle of humerus → below the axilla → surround the scapula → neck (meeting with foot Tai yang urinary bladder channel) → behind ear → enter the ear → above the auricle → beneath the mandible → outer canthus and temple → around teeth → angle or the natural hairline.

Diagnostic posture:
- Prone posture: (1) Arm pronation, (2) behind arm (palpating), and (3) sinus area.
- Supine posture: (1) Arm supination and (2) triceps (palpating).
- Standing posture: Raise arm with all different directions of hands.

Diagnostic points: Skin color, depression, armpit wrinkle, pressure on head, ear area wrinkle, facial muscles, acne, muscle tension, the location of scapular, skin tension.

Related muscles: Flexor carpi ulnaris, triceps brachii (long head), teres minor, infraspinatus, subscapularis, rhomboids, levator scapular, splenius capitis, auricularis (posterior, superior, anterior) muscles, masseter muscle, between the frontal belly of epicranius muscle and temporal fascia.

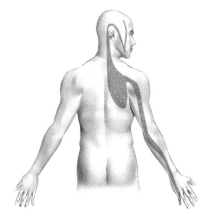

FIGURE 7.2
Hand Tai yang small intestine muscle.

Hand Shao Yang San Jiao (Triple Burner) Meridian Flow (Figure 7.3)

Pathway:
- Fourth finger → wrist → forearm → olecranon elbow → shoulder → neck (meeting with arm Tai yang small intestine meridian) → ear to outer canthus → temple.
- Another branch of fourth finger → wrist → forearm → olecranon elbow → shoulder → neck (meeting with arm Tai yang small intestine meridian) → mandible → base of the tongue.

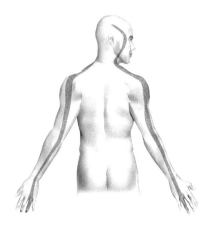 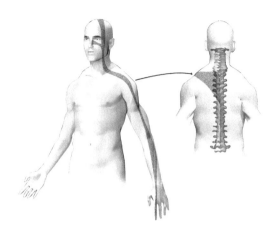

FIGURE 7.3
Hand Shao yang San Jiao muscle meridian.

FIGURE 7.4
Hand Yang Ming large intestine muscle meridian flow.

Diagnostic posture:
- Lying on side: Pull arm downward and check the neck muscle and heads of deltoid muscle balance.
- Standing posture: Palpate the neck muscle to the ear.

Diagnostic points: Skin color, depression, armpit wrinkle, pressure on head, facial and neck congestion.

Related muscles: Extensor digitorum, triceps brachii (lateral head), deltoid muscle, supraspinatus, levator scapular, splenius capitis, masseter muscle, temporalis muscle, hyoglossus muscle.

Hand Yang Ming Large Intestine Meridian Flow (Figure 7.4)

Pathway:
- Index finger → wrist → forearm → elbow → shoulder → capular → spine.
- Index finger → wrist → forearm → elbow → shoulder or neck (meeting with hand Tai yang small intestine meridian) → side of nose.
- Index finger → wrist → forearm → elbow → shoulder or neck (meeting with hand Tai yang small intestine meridian) → mandible or head.

Diagnostic posture:
- Supine posture: (1) Pronate arm toward abdomen, and with (2) hands up on head, check the shoulder.
- Prone posture: Palpate the upper thoracic spine area.
- Standing posture: Check the posture (kyphosis).

Diagnostic points: Skin color, depression, armpit wrinkle, muscle tightness, facial muscles.

Related muscles: Extensor carpi radialis, supinator, deltoid muscle, trapezius, levator scapular, splenius capitis, masseter muscle, zygomaticus.

Three Hand Yin Meridians

The three hand yin meridians are frequently used in type M1 yin syndrome treatment, diagnosis, and prognosis. The following represent the clinical syndrome:

- Upper arm and shoulder area congestion (upper fat tissue congestion)
- Armpit and back of arm congestion

- Protruding shape of chest area
- Pectoralis muscle tightness
- Shortness of breath
- Chest tightness
- Easily feeling sad
- After eating, bloating and feeling full in epigastric area
- Abdominal distension

Hand Tai Yin Lung Muscle Meridian Flow (Figure 7.5)

Pathway: Thumb → thenar eminence → wrist at pulse → forearm or elbow → thoracic cavity (enter chest area below the axillar) → front of clavicle → diaphragm.

Diagnostic posture: Supine posture: Arms supinate and check the clavicle level.

Diagnostic points: Skin color, depression, armpit wrinkle, muscle tightness, blood vessel, sensitivity to touch, breathing motion (abdominal and thoracic).

Related muscles: Thenar muscles, brachioradialis, biceps brachii muscle, pectoralis major muscle, pectoralis minor muscle, serratus anterior, intercostal muscle.

Hand Jue Yin Pericardium Muscle Meridian Flow (Figure 7.6)

Pathway: Medial finger (palmar) → hand Tai yin muscle meridian → medial elbow → axilla → spreading rib (front and back) → diaphragm.

Diagnostic posture: Supine posture: (1) With arm supinate, check the line of muscles; (2) raise arm and check the armpit for swelling or mass; and (3) check rib cage structure.

Diagnostic points: Skin color, depression, armpit wrinkle, muscle tightness, blood vessel, sensitivity to touch,

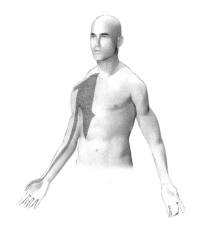

FIGURE 7.5
Hand Tai yin lung muscle meridian.

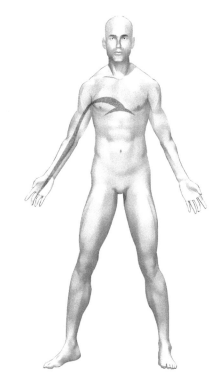

FIGURE 7.6
Hand Jue yin pericardium muscle meridian.

and breathing motion (abdominal and thoracic).

Related muscles: Flexor digitorum, brachioradialis, biceps brachii muscle, serratus anterior, intercostal muscle, diaphragm.

Hand Shao Yin Heart Meridian Flow (Figure 7.7)

Pathway: Little finger → pisiform bone → medial elbow → thoracic cavity or axillar → hand Tai yin muscle meridian or breast → diaphragm → umbilicus.

Diagnostic posture: Supine posture: (1) With arm supinate, check the armpit, and (2) check the midline of the chest and upper abdominal area.

Diagnostic points: Skin color, depression, armpit wrinkle, muscle tightness, blood vessel, sensitivity of touch, xiphoidal area mass.

Related muscles: Flexor digitorum, biceps brachii muscle, pectoralis major muscle, pectoralis minor muscle, serratus anterior, intercostal muscle, diaphragm, median umbilical ligament.

Hand Yin Muscle Meridian Reference

Breathing Primary Muscle: Diaphragm

The diaphragm controls

- Breathing
- Lymphatic fluid transfer
- Moving while asleep

The diaphragm is the major muscle of inspiration and accounts for approximately 70% of the inhaled tidal volume in normal people. Contraction of the diaphragm results in a downward motion of the muscle, as well as outward and upward movement of the ribs through the zone of apposition.

Intercostal Muscles

The intercostal muscles are located between the ribs, with three layers running in different directions. They include the external, internal, and innermost transverse muscles that contain the blood vessels and nerves. The artery, vein, and nerve are on the lower edge of each rib. A prolonged sitting posture, intestinal fatty tissue congestion, or diaphragm sprain make the intercostal space narrow and restrict movement.

Breathing Secondary Muscle

This comprises

- Sternocleidomastoid
- Serratus posterior
- Levatores costarum

The rib cage is the bony group structure connecting in the front at the sternum and at the back to the spine. It has the important

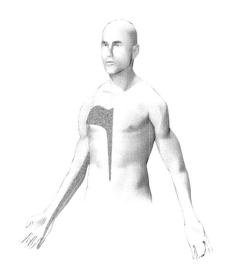

FIGURE 7.7
Hand Shao yin heart muscle meridian.

function of protecting major organs, adjusting the flexibility of organ structures, and facilitating respiration in the diaphragm. The rib cage has more than 80 joints, and the sternum and ribs are connected on a flexible costal cartilage. Mobilizing the rib cage indirectly aids cardiac and respiratory function. During respiration, the rib cage moves forward and upward, similar to a bucket handle motion. Several upper thoracic muscles are involved in mobilizing the rib cage:

- Scalenes: Pulls ribs 2 and 3
- Sternocleidomastoid muscle (SCM): Sternum
- Serratus anterior: Ribs 7–10
- Pectoralis minor: Ribs 3–5
- Pectoralis major: Ribs 6–8
- Back muscle
- Levatores costarum: Ribs 1–4

The SCM connects to the sternum, clavicle, and mastoid process. This muscle has the action of elevating the first rib and sternum to breathe. The sternomastoids are probably the most important accessory muscles of inspiration, and their participation in breathing with dyspnea is a well-known clinical observation.

Abdominal Muscles

The abdominal muscles (rectus abdominis, internal oblique, external oblique, and transverse abdominis) serve a number of functions in respiration, mainly assisting expiration, but they can also function in inspiration (Figure 7.8). The internal and external obliques and the transversus abdominis result in an inward movement of the abdominal wall that displaces the diaphragm upward into the thoracic cavity and assists exhalation. The rectus abdominis and the internal and external obliques

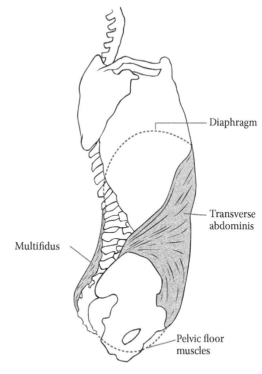

FIGURE 7.8
Diaphragm and abdominal muscle.

pull the lower rib cage caudally and thereby increase pleural pressure and exhalation. The abdominal muscles may also play a minor role in inspiration.

Other Breathing Muscles

These comprise

- Muscles attached to the upper extremity of the body
- Pectoralis major and minor muscles, which lie anteriorly and superficially
- Posterior superficial musculature, which includes the trapezius and latissimus dorsi
- Deep muscles, which include the serratus anterior and posterior, the levatores, and the major and minor rhomboids

These superficial and deep muscles help hold the scapulae to the chest wall.

In respiratory distress, the deltoid, pectoralis, and latissimus dorsi muscles form a tertiary system for ventilator assistance through fixation of the upper extremities.

Three Foot Yang Meridians

The three foot yang meridians are used in treatment of types M2 and T.

Clinical Syndrome

- Back pain radiating to legs or upper back and shoulder
- Knee pain when cold
- Sudden weight gain
- Skin allergy on eye and facial area
- Foot pain
- Love handles (hard to distinguish waist and hip area)
- Feeling cold or hot
- Sweat easily or not much sweat
- Lordosis
- Big belly
- Body swollen or fat distribution relatively even on entire body area
- Feeling of emptiness, depression and anxiety, aggression

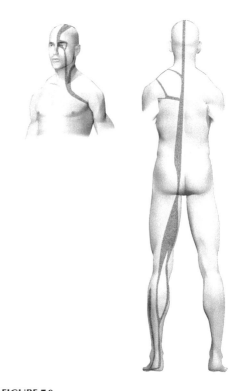

FIGURE 7.9
Foot Tai yang urinary bladder muscle meridian.

Foot Tai Yang Urinary Bladder Meridian Flow (Figure 7.9)

Pathway: Little toe → external malleolus → knee → heel → popliteal fossa → gastrocnemius muscle area → gluteus region → spine and nape → root of tongue → occipital bone → nose bridge → eye → side of below nose.

Little toe → external malleolus → knee → heel → popliteal fossa → gastrocnemius muscle area → gluteus region → spine and nape → posterior axillary fold → large intestine major meridian Li15 (anterior–inferior to the acromion, on the upper portion of M. deltoideus) → chest below axilla → supraclavicular fossa → GB12 major meridian point area (on the head, posterior to the auricle, in the depression posterior and inferior to the mastoid process) behind ear.

Diagnostic posture:
1. Pronate posture: Arm pronate, and check the neck.
2. Supinate posture: Check the foot direction.
3. Standing posture: Shoes, neck bending.

Diagnostic points: Skin color, depression, muscle tightness, blood vessel, swollen spot, and the circular range of motion on ankle, waist–hip line, and neck.

Related muscles: Gastrocnemius, soleus muscle, biceps femoris, semitendinosus, tendon area of the gluteus muscle, multifidus, spinalis muscle, between the latissimus dorsi muscle and trapezius, between pectoralis major and deltoid muscle, between trapezius and SCM muscle, semispinalis capitis muscle, occipital and frontal belly of epicarnius muscle, scalp, orbicularis muscle.

Foot Shao Yang Gallbladder Meridian Flow (Figure 7.10)

Pathway: Fourth toe → external malleolus → lateral knee → fibular and thigh → major meridian point ST 32 (on the anterior side of the thigh and on the line connecting the anteriosuperior iliac spine and the superiolateral corner of the patella, three cm above this corner) → sacrum → anterior axillar → breast region or clavicle bone → clavicle area (meet with foot Tai yang urinary bladder channel) → behind ear or temple → vertex → cheek, nose, or outer canthus.

Diagnostic posture:
- Side bending posture: (1) Pulling the leg to check the aligned muscle, and (2) pulling up the arm to check congestion of the armpit area.
- Standing and sitting posture: Head tilted, unstable facial muscle movement check, and temporal artery check.

Diagnostic points: Skin color, depression, armpit wrinkle, muscle tightness, blood vessel, sensitivity to touch, alignment with muscles, and passive range of motion (legs and arms).

Related muscles: Extensor digitorum longus, fiburalis longus, tensor fascia latae, gluteus muscle, frontal edge of the latissimus dorsi muscle, between the pectoralis major and latissimus dorsi muscle, edge of the trapezius muscle, occipital belly of the epicarnius muscle, auricularis posterior muscle, temporalis muscle, orbicularis oculi muscle.

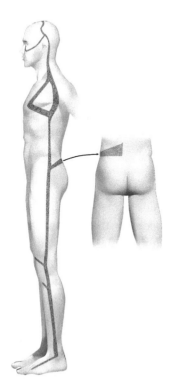

FIGURE 7.10
Foot Shao yang gallbladder muscle meridian.

Foot Yang Ming Stomach Meridian Flow (Figure 7.11)

Pathway: Second, third, fourth toes → lateral legs → knee → across the hip → lower rib → spine.

Second, third, fourth toes → lateral legs → fibular → foot Shao yang gallbladder channel → thigh → pelvic or reproductive area → abdomen or chest → clavicle → neck or mouth → nose → eye or foot Tai yang urinary bladder channel → jaw or face → ear.

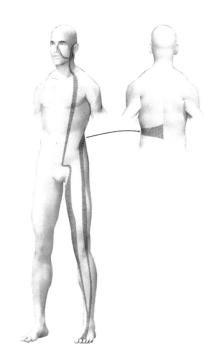

FIGURE 7.11
Foot Yang Ming stomach muscle meridian.

Diagnostic posture:
- Supine posture: (1) Bending the leg to check the aligned muscle, (2) ankle flexion and extension, and (3) neck congestion and facial expression.
- Standing posture: Abdominal shape and side congestion.
- Side bending: Check between the hip and rib bone.

Diagnostic points: Skin color, depression, muscle tightness, lower abdominal pressure, protruding rib cage, clavicle area congestion, neck muscles, facial expression, blood vessel, sensitivity to touch, acne.

Related muscles: Extensor digitorum longus, tibialis anterior muscle, quadriceps femoris muscle, adductor longus muscle, latissimus dorsi, transverse abdominis, rectus abdominis, oblique muscles, pectoral muscles, SCM, masseter muscle, orbicularis oris muscle, orbicularis (omit) muscle.

Three Foot Yin Meridians

For six body types treatment, the three foot yin meridians are closely related to type M3.

Clinical Syndrome

- Gynecology problem, male reproductive problem
- Lower extremities vein problem (varicose veins, spider veins)
- Bending forward from the midback posture or neck straightened
- Ankylosing spondylitis
- Urinary incontinence
- Occipital headache
- Toe and heel problem
- Fearful and afraid

Foot Tai Yin Spleen Muscle Meridian Flow (Figure 7.12)

Pathway: Big toe (medial) → internal malleolus → medial side of knee → medical thigh → hip or reproductive area → abdomen or umbilicus → ribs or chest → spine.

Diagnostic posture:
- Supine posture: (1) Palpate alongside of meridian, (2) check the tension or depression on the lower abdominal area, and (3) check bunion and foot status.
- Prone posture: Midback area fatty tissue accumulation or deep skin wrinkle from spine to side of rib.

Diagnostic points: Skin temperature, depression, skin tightness, muscle tightness, blood vessel, sensitivity to touch, the direction of umbilicus (pulled downward or upward), midback spine.

Muscle Meridian Therapy and Skin Cutaneous Therapy • 135

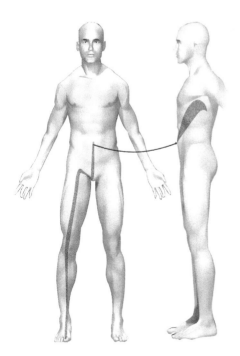

FIGURE 7.12
Foot Tai yin spleen muscle meridian.

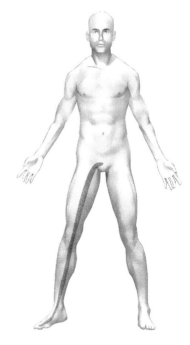

FIGURE 7.13
Foot Jue yin liver muscle meridian.

Related muscles and ligaments: Extensor hallucis longus, between the medial edge of the soleus and gastrocnemius muscle and tibialis bone, vastus medialis, adductor longus, semimembranosus, gracilis muscle, inguinal ligament, pyramidalis muscle, falciform ligament, peritoneum, serratus posterior inferior muscle.

Foot Jue Yin Liver Meridian Flow (Figure 7.13)

Pathway: Big toe → internal malleolus → medial tibia → inside of knee → medial thigh → genitals.

Diagnostic posture:
- Standing posture: Check the congestion on medial anterior area of the thigh.
- Supine posture: Palpate the meridian medial side of the knee.

Diagnostic points: Swollen inner thigh area and lower back, the gap between knees, pressure sensitivity on meridian.

Related muscles: Extensor hallucis longus, between the medial edge of the soleus and gastrocnemius muscle and tibialis bone, vastus medialis, adductor longus, semimembranosus, gracilis muscle, pubic tubercle.

Foot Shao Yin Kidney Meridian Flow (Figure 7.14)

Pathway: Beneath little toe → meeting with foot Tai yin spleen muscle meridian → internal malleolus → heel→ foot Tai yang urinary bladder meridian → lower or medial knee → foot Tai yin spleen muscle meridian or thigh area → genital region → side of spine → nape of neck → occipital bone → foot Tai yang urinary bladder channel.

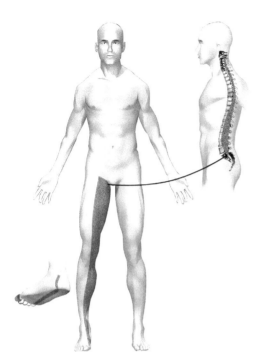

FIGURE 7.14
Foot Shao yin kidney muscle meridian.

Diagnostic posture:
- Standing posture: (1) Palpate alongside the meridian, (2) check the tension or depression on the lower abdominal area, (3) palpate on the abdomen deeply, and (4) check back spine posture.
- Supinate posture: Ankle direction.
- Pronate posture: (1) Feet, (2) blood vessel, (3) spine structure, and (4) occiput.

Diagnostic points: Sole fat cushion, dry skin, depression, skin color, skin tightness, blood vessel, spine curvature, neck congestion (occiput area).

Related muscles: Flexor digitorum brevis, extensor hallucis longus, between the medial edge of the soleus and gastrocnemius muscle and tibialis bone, hip adductor muscles (adductor brevis, adductor longus, adductor magnus, adductor minimus), levator ani muscle, rectococcygeus muscle, anterior sacrococcygeal ligament, anterior longitudinal ligament.

CUTANEOUS MERIDIAN

The cutaneous meridian is a connective system in TCM. It connects the external surface of the body to the internal organs. Furthermore, it connects the upper and lower body as well as the extremities to the trunk. It is the body surface area within which Qi and blood flow.

In Chapter 56 of the ancient medical classic *Plain Question*, the text states that the cutaneous regions are the part of the meridian system located in the superficial layers of the body and are marked by regular meridians.

In traditional Chinese medicine, whenever meridian and organ systems are explained, the Qi, blood flow, and balance are emphasized from the very first sentence. The meridian system is accredited from the origin of medicine, and is based on the observations and experiences of the living human body, not from cadaver anatomy.

It is not just manifested from a skin or dermatological aspect. The meridian system is unlike Western medicine, which classifies body systems according to skeletal, muscular, circulatory, digestive, urinary, nervous, reproductive, lymphatic, endocrine, and respiratory systems. Recently, many researchers have identified the skin as an important immune system of the body.

Since the cutaneous meridian is connected to internal organisms, external pathogenic factors can penetrate to the internal organs through this meridian. Moreover, an internal disorder can be manifested to the cutaneous meridian region if not treated.

Clinically, observation of the skin area is helpful in finding the problem area and the root of the disorder.

Function of Skin

In TCM, the cutaneous skin has a close relationship with lung Qi, which protects organisms from exterior pathogenic factors. The lung Qi circulates through and warms the skin. Thus, skin color change is related to the status of internal organs.

Bluish purple indicates local pain, a dark color indicates blockage from obstruction, yellow and red are signs of heat, and a pale complexion is due to cold.

The functions of the skin (integumentary) system are protection, body temperature regulation, blood reservoir, and excretion. Skin also provides tactility, which is the sense of touch, and produces vitamin D, which is needed for proper body functions.

The skin regulates body temperature by causing the peripheral blood vessels to contract or dilate. If the body temperature is elevated, blood vessels dilate to allow for evaporation, and so lower body temperature as sweat is released. If the body is cold, the blood vessels contract in the dermis area in order to retain body heat. This results in a change of complexion depending on the interior or exterior temperature. Contracted blood vessels result in a bluish pale facial complexion; dilated blood vessels cause facial complexion to turn a pinkish red.

Purple or darkish gray color is linked to venous insufficiency. In fact, an important role of the skin is as a blood reservoir, storing 8%–10% of the total blood. When you are in a healthy state, blood remains in the peripheral blood vessels, distributes nutrients and oxygen to cells, and removes waste products from cells. However, when you are stressed, your autonomic nervous system restricts the blood vessels. If you are in a state of chronic tension or stress, your skin will become dry and darker in color.

Since the skin is the first layer of exposure to hot or cold exterior conditions, it is related to thyroid function, which controls your body's temperature. If chronic skin and muscle tension are not resolved, your core temperature is reduced and may result in a hormone imbalance.

Cases have shown the relationship between the thyroid and the skin. A problem with the structure of the thyroid results in a goiter, which can restrict the airway and cause weakening of the breathing muscles. Again, a weakened breathing muscle cannot provide a good source of nutrients and oxygen to the distal peripheral area, which is the skin. This results in a weakening of the skin and a weakening of the body's protection system. Body systems influence each other and are involved with the structural function. We need to focus more on a systemic loop, with regard to symptoms and signs, rather than trying to clear the symptoms.

Six Body Types and Skin

Diagnosis for the Skin Meridian

For the six body types, skin is an important guideline for diagnosis and assessment for developing a treatment plan, as the condition of the skin differs according to internal systemic conditions and the local problems. For example, if a skin disorder occurs on the arm, it can immediately rule out at least two different etiologic hypotheses. One is the local congestion from tension stress due to lengthened muscle inflammation, and the other is from body temperature imbalances due to chronic stress-induced conditions. Even though psoriasis has been diagnosed, the treatment will differ depending on the root of the skin disorder. For this, an entire and detailed diagnostic process should be followed, which examines not just the depth of disease, but also other organ issues, body types, and lifestyle.

The skin meridian connects the skin to the entire body, allowing each system to communicate, protect, and maintain the homeostatic system with one another.

Treatment of the Skin Meridian

Prognosis

In an acupuncture clinic setting, a cutaneous needle is used for superficial stimulation. Medicinal ointment and a patch can be used on the area that correlates with the internal organ. Furthermore, infrared heat and moxibustion are used as hyperthermal treatment methods of meridian therapy.

The function of moxibustion is to stimulate the skin's immune system.

For a six body types treatment setting, I use moxa oil and a tongue depressor as treatment tools in cutaneous meridian therapy.

Skin Meridian

1. Tai yang cutaneous meridian (urinary bladder and small intestine)
2. Shao yang cutaneous meridian (gallbladder and San Jiao)
3. Yang Ming cutaneous meridian (stomach and large intestine)
4. Tai yin cutaneous meridian (spleen and lung)
5. Jue yin cutaneous meridian (liver and pericardium)
6. Shao yin cutaneous meridian (kidney and heart)

Clinical Syndrome

The cutaneous meridian has 12 different pathways and regions, followed by 12 primary meridians. However, patterns of clinical observation indicate that people have similar superficial conditions, such as body fluids or fat deposits, depending on the symptoms and signs. I have classified six patterns in total.

Tai Yang Cutaneous Meridian Pattern (Figure 7.15)

This condition is displayed when the individual has been in a state of intense stress, physically or mentally. In fact, the person can feel a pulsation on his back when he works hard or is sitting for an extended

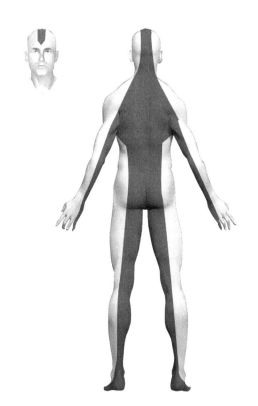

FIGURE 7.15
Tai yang cutaneous meridian.

period. After intense working periods, the neck to lower back begins to ache and a feeling a tightness affects all body movement. This type is also associated with heat sensitivity. Movement will be energetic and pronounced.

Skin condition: Dark color, acne, tense feeling upon palpation, body hair; if severe, pores and lumps are pronounced.

Shao Yang Cutaneous Meridian Pattern (Figure 7.16)

This condition usually develops after shock and chronic stress situations, such as trauma, surgery, family issues, and weakness following chronic illness. This type is associated with a short attention span, excessive thirst, fatigue, and digestion problems. The side of the body has congestion with heat signs.

Skin condition: Skin allergy, goose bumps following stimulation, rough "chicken skin" on arms, eczema, and psoriasis.

Yang Ming Cutaneous Meridian Pattern (Figure 7.17)

This meridian's pathogenic symptoms are caused by an internally active inflammatory status. Swelling and itching occur, or skin tightness accompanied by symptoms of heartburn. Food poisoning, drinking alcohol, food allergies, chronic indigestion, and PMS can result.

Skin condition: Acne, skin redness, swollen acute fat tissue deposit, itching, and dark spots.

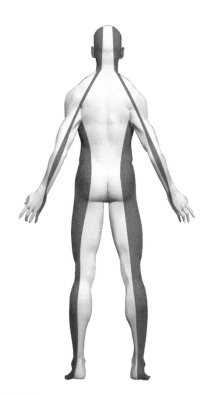

FIGURE 7.16
Shao yang cutaneous meridian.

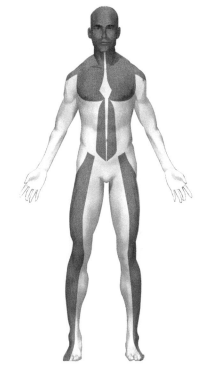

FIGURE 7.17
Yang Ming cutaneous meridian.

Tai Yin Cutaneous Meridian Pattern (Figure 7.18)

This type of pathogenic incident results from extremity trauma, infections, or inflammation. It is usually accompanied by lymphatic congestion and stretch marks. In such cases, it is necessary to inquire about the medical history regarding childhood incidents involving extremities or severe infection around lymph nodes. This condition is also accompanied by a body temperature imbalance, for example, feeling cold due to muscle weakness.

Skin condition: Stretch marks (brown color), no flexibility of skin, dark color, sweat pores are exposed and appear swollen.

Jue Yin Cutaneous Meridian Pattern (Figure 7.19)

This area of the skin is related to breathing and circulation problems. The most common type of case is caused by gynecologic surgery and chronic pain symptoms. Initial stages of pathogens in the Jue yin cutaneous meridian are presented as swelling or dampness on the medial thigh and under the breast area, whereas the hand and feet distal skin is shown to have a lack of fatty cushioning and is thin and weak. Acne and discharge occur if a severe lymph congestion condition is prevalent due to skin allergy itching on the trunk and medial thigh area. In the chronic stage, the area of

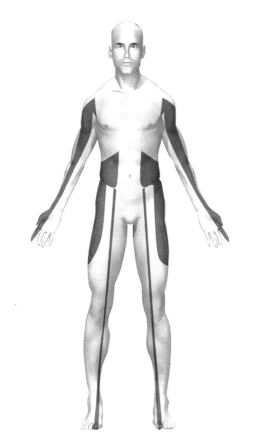

FIGURE 7.18
Tai yin cutaneous meridian.

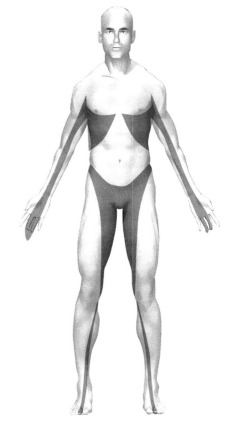

FIGURE 7.19
Jue yin cutaneous meridian.

skin will display fatty tissue congestion and will be thick, and the mass of skin and fat in the area can be grabbed. It results in restriction of movement beneath the muscles. It is also related to peripheral neuropathy and peripheral blood vessel problems.

Skin condition: Skin tightness, wet and oily to the touch, fat deposits, thickness of skin, discoloration, abnormal skin temperature, wrinkles.

Shao Yin Cutaneous Meridian Pattern (Figure 7.20)

The Shao yin cutaneous meridian is related to chronic breathing and circulation problems due to spinal problems. In clinical observation, it is accompanied by rib cage deformities such as protruding ribs or protruding sternum and raised ribs. Chronic heart and lung disorder may result from this condition. The area of the Shao yin cutaneous meridian will display spider veins or dry skin and depression rather than swelling.

Skin condition: Small veins, red spots, easily bruised, dry skin.

Myotome and Dermatome

While cutaneous meridians are used for diagnosis and treatment of connecting internal organs, the dermatome and myotome are more specifically differentiated on a sectional anatomy chart.

These nerve plexus form two sets of branches from the spine; one is from C5 to T2, and the other from T12 to S1. These two areas are near the parasympathetic nerve arising areas.

A dermatome is a sensory region of skin innervated by a single nerve root and by its corresponding spinal nerve, and myatome is a muscle area innervated by a single nerve root.

Dermatomes are useful to help localize neurologic levels, particularly in radiculopathy. Effacement or encroachment of a spinal nerve may or may not exhibit symptoms in the dermatomic area covered by the compressed nerve roots, in addition to weakness, or deep tendon reflex loss.

Common dermatomal levels are

- C5: Shoulder
- C6: Lateral arm and fingers 1 and 2
- C7: Middle finger
- C8: Fingers 4 and 5
- L4: Anteromedial shin
- L5: Anterolateral shin, dorsum of foot to big toe
- S1: Toe, lateral foot, sole, and calf

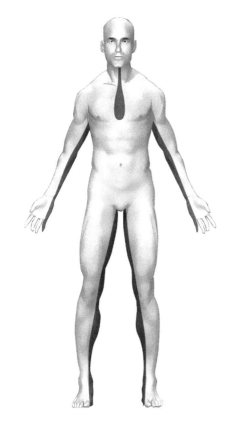

FIGURE 7.20
Shao yin cutaneous meridian.

The arm muscles, the biceps brachii, and the deltoid are innervated by C5 and C6. The biceps brachii is innervated by C5 and C6, but the deltoid muscle is innervated by C5. This group of muscles is used to test for shoulder abduction.

Neurologic level C6: The biceps brachii is innervated by C5 and C6. C6 also innervates the most powerful wrist extensors, carpi radialis longus and brevis, which carry out radial extension.

Neurologic level C7: The muscles found within this myotomal pattern are the triceps and wrist flexors. The triceps muscle primarily controls elbow extension.

Neurologic level C8: The muscles within this myotomal pattern are finger flexors—flexor digitorum superficialis, flexor digitorum profundus, and the lumbricals.

Neurologic level T1: The muscles within this myotomal pattern are those involved in finger abduction (dorsal interossei and abductor digiti minimi) and adduction (palmar interossei).

Neurologic levels T12–L3: The muscles within this myotomal pattern are the iliopsoas, quadriceps, and adductors. Because this myotomal pattern includes multiple muscle groups, an injury to this nerve root level can be more easily evaluated by sensory testing of the dermatomal patterns.

Neurologic level L4: The muscle predominantly innervated at this root nerve level is the tibialis anterior, which is responsible for dorsiflexion.

Neurologic level L5: The muscles within this myotome are the extensor hallucis longus (big toe extensor) and extensor digitorum (heel walk).

Neurologic level S1: The muscles within this myotome are the peroneus longus (eversion) and peroneus brevis (eversion). Dermatome and myotome are useful diagnostic maps, as well as treatment guides. In my clinic, I use moxa oil and a tongue depressor with guided maps for treating cutaneous meridians.

8

Treatment Methods

CLINICAL SETTING

Muscle Meridian Acupuncture Technique

The muscle meridian acupuncture technique is used for treating disorders or misaligned skeletal muscles, tendons, and ligaments according to the muscle meridians. This method requires manipulating the needle while continually observing the condition of motion when targeting a meridian area. It is aimed at correcting muscle imbalance as well as treating tissue within the muscle and tendon structures. The treatment targets both stretched (lengthened) muscle and contracted (shortened) muscle areas and the space between the muscles.

Since a muscle meridian covers the surface dimensions of the entire body, the treatment unit is the area rather than the point. Furthermore, acupuncture needling is different from the point needle in that it waits for Qi acquisition. Once the needle is inserted into the problem area, it is moved further forward or backward along the tension line, hardened mass, or surface of contracted muscle fibers for several seconds, and then the needle is removed immediately.

Patients may feel a heavy, distended, sharp, or burning pain, depending on their internal symptoms. A twitching sensation occurs regardless of the trigger point or soft tissue stimulated during the treatment session.

Like other meridian treatments, of course, the entire diagnosis assessment is important for establishing a treatment plan, but the muscle meridian technique emphasizes the practitioner's objective observations and palpations. In order to gain information on the internal condition of a patient, the skin and subcutaneous area between the muscle and the skin plays a crucial role in determining the current and past condition. The depth of skin to the muscle, the status of subcutaneous parts, the skin surface temperature, and a wrinkle or spot on the skin all form part of the objective focus for muscle meridian acupuncture techniques.

The observation of a patient's condition begins as he or she walks in the door. Observations are made even while the patient stands, sits, drinks

143

tea, opens the door, lies down, and so forth. All movements and motions can be diagnostic clues. Finger and wrist tension, standing habits, and mouth movements are also important diagnostic standards. The practitioner will understand any restrictions, abnormal motions, and actions relating to the patient's unintentional movements.

Childhood trauma, surgeries, scar tissue, or abnormal body depression and wrinkles can be the first target areas to treat for muscle meridian imbalances. Therefore, a detailed observation and history is recommended.

The practitioner asks questions regarding the primary problem and concerns, and then begins to determine whether there are any discolorations and wrinkles on the surface of the skin before proceeding to palpate along the muscle meridian with two left fingers. This enables the practitioner to check the pressure between the skin and muscle areas. The applied pressure should be gentle, using two fingers with an approximately 3-centimeter gap between the fingers. While pressing the skin alongside the problem area, the internal wrinkle can be observed, which indicates the presence of internal tissue adhesion. This is the point at which the needle is inserted when treating lengthened muscle fibers.

Summary of the Muscle Meridian Technique

- The treatment is aimed at the entire area, at the tensioned lines, or between the depth of the skin and muscle, not just the point.
- The objective observation is more important than local symptoms, so thorough diagnosis is required prior to the treatment plan.

- The treatment must begin at the weak muscle, stretched muscle area, body wrinkle line, or congested area.
- The needle is not kept in one spot, but the practitioner will manipulate the needle several times as it is inserted.
- The motion or condition of the needling area is checked frequently during treatment.

Cupping

Cupping is an ancient technique used in many cultures; it entails the use of a special cup applied to the skin and held in place by suction. The suction draws superficial tissue into the cup, which may be either left in place or moved along the body.

Cupping brings fresh blood to the area and helps improve circulation. The negative pressure of cupping increases local vascularity and oxygenation of tissues and eliminates edema fluid, exudate, extraverted blood, and bacteria.

Traditional cupping, sometimes referred to as fire cupping, uses heat to create a vacuum like suction inside of the glass cup. In modern times, cups that use a small pump to create suction have also been introduced, and the cup materials are varied. Korean traditional medicine doctors use automated cupping sets that are operated by electric pumps to release and suck the air in order to produce a massage effect. This also helps to remove excess lymphatic fluids.

Most patients feel relaxed and light after a cupping treatment. However, cupping therapy has several cautions and contraindications.

Contraindications of Cupping Therapy

- Skin ulcer
- Edema

- Not for use on large blood vessels
- High fever and convulsions
- In abdominal and sacral regions of pregnant woman
- If the patient suffers from hemophilia (bleeds easily)

Cupping therapy helps to move excess lymphatic fluids in the body, which would leave one to assume that it is beneficial for edema conditions. Interestingly, one of cupping therapy's contraindications is edema. Applying even a single session of cupping therapy for edema is not recommended, as it may worsen the condition. Without a doubt, cupping can help remove cold dampness, diminish swelling, and relieve pain if the treatment is carried out in the right way. However, it is not recommended to use cupping therapy as a home remedy.

Licensed acupuncturists practice several modalities to treat the conditions according to the treatment plan assessments. Cupping therapy is usually used in hyperemia conditions or after another modality has been used. In instances, if there is lack of heat sign or venous congestion, the cupping therapy should be applied cautiously.

The difference between edema and swelling depends on the artery and venous systems involved. The symptoms may seem similar because both include locally increased blood volumes.

Hyperemia is the active process of arteriolar dilation caused by inflammation or swelling of skeletal muscles during exercise. The affected tissue turns red from the oxygenated blood. Congestion is the passive systematic process known as cyanosis, in which the congested tissues are dusky and bluish in color. It is caused by cardiac failure or venous obstruction and gives rise to edema in tissue as a result of deoxygenated

hemoglobin. Again, caution must be exercised when treating this condition with cupping therapy.

After dermal needling or moxa oil scraping when treating the six body types, I use an automated motor suction cupping method in my clinic for various techniques. Since cupping applies negative pressure to suppressed or temporarily congested areas, acupressure can be applied to areas with the opposite condition in order to obtain a balance.

For example, the upper back displays heat symptoms and peripheral blood vessel congestion; the lower back presents with a cold swelling condition. I apply a cupping set on the upper back muscle area (negative pressure), followed by scraping with moxa oil for a mild positive pressure stimulation.

Cupping is frequently used on hematoma on distal extremities due to trauma, such as a sprained ankle. The superficial bloodletting technique is combined with wet-cupping therapy, which is different from regular cupping therapy (dry cupping).

Negative-pressure wound therapy (NPWT) is practiced in modern medical clinics. It is a therapeutic technique using a vacuum dressing to promote healing. It is also used in hospital settings to promote the healing of acute and chronic wounds, partial-thickness burns, diabetic and mild pressure ulcers, and skin grafts.

Moxa Oil and Gua Sha

Moxa oil is made from mugwort, a common weed originating in eastern Europe and western Asia, but now found in many parts of the world. Its Latin name, *Artemisia vulgaris*, distinguishes it from the many other species of *Artemisia* grown and used around the world. *Artemisia princeps, Artemisia montana*, and *Artemisia iwayomogi* are frequently used as a good-quality moxibustion floss in Japan, and medicinal mugwort (as yet unspecified, shaped like lion's foot dorsum) is cultivated in Korea and is widely known as a strong medicinal herb.

Korea is well known as the country of fermented food, such as kimchi, and its inhabitants eat substantial quantities of garlic. Korean ancestors placed emphasis on hygiene of the external and internal body conditions and maintaining a clean environment. In 2333 B.C., the first Korean kingdom was founded in northern China and the Korean peninsula, according to the Dangun Wanggeom legend, and garlic and mugwort were introduced as spiritual Korean herbs.

Mugwort intended for medicinal purposes should first be dried for at least three years, and special care needs to be taken; otherwise, toxic substances are present that can affect neurologic functions in the body.

Moxibustion is used as a hyperthermal therapeutic method on the skin to treat cold symptoms and immune deficiencies. Hyperthermal methods are the oldest known therapy, originating from the same era when the first humans began using fire. Well-dried weeds or plant flosses generate a higher heat temperature and penetrate deeper into body parts. The penetrating heat results in muscle relaxation and improves circulation.

The ancient experiences were handed down and developed into one of the most important treatment methods, moxibustion. Most traditional Chinese and Korean medicinal acupuncture books are entitled *Acupuncture and Moxibustion*.

In my clinic, I use moxa oil and a tongue depressor as the treatment method of the six body types. As I treat skin, muscles, and subcutaneous areas, instant local peripheral blood vessel dilation plays an important role in loosening and moving congested body fluids.

Hyperthermal Methods

Moxibustion

Moxibustion is a hyperthermal treatment method that is carried out by applying a burning herb in various ways to appropriate points or large surfaces on the body. Moxibustion can be used alone as a primary therapy or in combination with acupuncture. Bian Que of the spring and autumn period (770–476 B.C.), the well-known doctor in China, mentioned a treatment method following the depth of pathogenic factors in the body. His statement, "first acupuncture, second moxibustion, third an herbal formula," has been translated in different ways, depending on the ideas and theories of the translator.

In the *Ling Shu* (*The Spiritual Pivot*) Chapter 73, "A disease that may not be treated by acupuncture may be treated by moxibustion." This supports a famous Japanese medicinal quote about moxibustion: "Moxa can treat anything that is difficult to cure." This method involves the burning of moxa (mugwort). The heat of the cauterization, as well as the properties of the moxa itself, serve to warm the Qi and blood in the channels, expel cold and dampness, restore yang, and in general, help regulate the organs and restore health. It is commonly used for gynecological problems and digestive and immune deficiency disorders. Mugwort has insecticidal, diuretic, and hemostatic properties. It has been widely used as a home remedy in various countries in Asia, especially Korea and Japan.

Although many studies and experiences show the effectiveness and safety of moxibustion in traditional Chinese medicine (TCM), few studies have tested moxibustion as a treatment of health conditions. Some of the evidence related to moxibustion is listed below:

- Moxibustion and hot flashes: Research showed that 14 sessions of moxibustion reduced the frequency and severity of hot flashes of 51 postmenopausal woman in 2009.
- Moxibustion and ulcerative colitis: A writer analyzed five clinical trials and determined that moxibustion possessed some benefits for people with ulcerative colitis.
- Moxibustion and breech birth: In 2005, scientists found insufficient evidence to support the use of moxibustion in correcting a breech presentation. Experienced TCM doctors recommend that this treatment be applied before 37 weeks for pregnancy for better results.

Ja-Hun

Ja-Hun (hyperthermal therapy for the urogenital and rectal area) is a treatment method handed down from ancient Asia. Ja-Hun does not just use heat for therapy alone, but also combines it with the well-known traditional Chinese medicinal herb, moxa (mugwort). Heat has long been recognized as an effective tool for pain management, muscle relaxation, and managing of hemorrhoids.

In the same way, heat is an appropriate method for relieving prostate problems in men. In addition, mugwort (also known as *Artemisia vulgaris* or Ai Ye, 艾) has long

been used as a folk remedy. It especially increases blood circulation to the pelvic area and uterus, and it warms the womb to help relieve menstrual pain and regulate cycles.

Ja-Hun therapy provides heat directly to the urogenital and anal canal, relaxing the muscles in the area and promoting venous circulation to encourage a natural healing process. In Korean cultures, Ja-Hun is not only a traditional medicine treatment method, but also "the wisdom gained from life." According to a Korean grandmother, "if you don't want to have gynecological problems, ignite on a gung yi [stove] and keep it burning all day." A gung yi is a fireplace for an ondol, which is underfloor heating that uses direct heat transfer from wood smoke to the underside of a thick stone floor. A traditional ondol was heated with mainly rice paddy straws, dried weeds, or any kind of dried firewood.

A woman's place, the kitchen, was also an important spot for sharing culture and educating younger ones. While preparing a meal for her family, a woman would sit in front of an a gung yi and absorb the natural heat therapy from it. An a gung yi's heat would be transferred to an ondol floor, which provided warmth to the family and so relaxed muscles during the night. Since Korean houses have been Westernized, it is not easy to find a traditional ondol in housing units. However, a Korean-style sauna, called a zzim jil bang (heat stone room sauna), is a popular place for families and friends to get together and relax and detoxify from the busy Korean lifestyle.

Gastrointestinal Resuscitation

Gastrointestinal resuscitation (GIR) is the process of reviving and reeducating the mechanical function of the gastrointestinal system with TCM methods such as acupuncture, cupping, moxibustion, and abdominal tension massage. GIR not only restores gastrointestinal functions, but also fosters emotional relaxation through improved abdominal breathing.

Our gut is connected to our brain and nervous system, as well as our hormonal system, major emotions, comfort and discomfort, and levels of anxiety or serenity. Traditional Chinese medicine teaches practitioners to focus first on the stomach and gut (middle Jiao) to get the Qi moving. Once the middle abdominal section is soft and has enough room for abdominal breathing, the Qi starts moving more smoothly through all body channels. It may not be easy for the abdomen to breathe for some, as they are influenced by habit, stress, body posture, or ailments.

GIR is an excellent noninvasive treatment for patients who have chronic distension, constipation, idiopathic back pain, and a cold abdomen. Abdominal tension is not always stressful, but it drives psychological tension from unpredictable incidents, similar to immobility in areas with limited maneuverability. This is because we spend an increasing amount of time sitting behind a desk typing on a keyboard, or typing on the small keypads of cellphones.

Many people spend too much time frozen in a tense, sitting position. This causes us to breathe less deeply with our chests, which exacerbates anxiety and stress. Shallow breathing can cause increased heart rate and muscle tension. Furthermore, simply overeating results in a distended belly, which results in a host of symptoms that will need therapy in the future if health is to be restored.

Benefits of GIR

- Loosening tension in the abdominal cavity
- Stretching restricted intestinal ligaments and soft tissues
- Warming accumulated adipose tissue
- Reducing inflammatory responses
- Aiding digestion, absorption, and peristaltic movement
- Facilitating abdominal breathing

CPR versus GIR

Cardiac pulmonary resuscitation (CPR) is a procedure that sends blood to the brain after a person has had a heart attack (or the heart has stopped beating for whatever reason) and is experiencing breathing difficulties. These life-threatening concerns are acute emergencies. CPR aids in circulating blood to the artery systems with the compression of the cardiac muscle in the thoracic cavity. GIR aids to bring blood from legs to heart with mild manipulating on lower abdominal area. It may help to prevent the vein obstruction in the pelvis or abdomen.

Acupressure

Characteristics of Acupressure Therapy

- Diagnosis and therapy combined
- Using only hands and fingers
- Fewer side effects
- Able to be applied to all age groups
- Treats the whole body

Acupressure was developed in Asia more than 5000 years ago. It is well known in Western culture as shiatsu, a Japanese form of acupressure. It is an ancient therapeutic body treatment using the fingers to gradually press acupuncture meridian points.

Like acupuncture treatment, acupressure is used to obtain an understanding of the condition of the entire body and to make an accurate observation. After understanding the symptoms and conditions, the practitioner will begin by pressing on the depressed spot alongside the meridians with two thumbs. Sometimes, a palm or hands are used to manipulate the problem area.

While using two thumbs to press the meridian points, a trained practitioner can detect abnormalities in the skin and muscles and body heat or cold congestion in local areas.

The practitioner's experience and sensitivity enable the control of the power dynamic applied to each point. This procedure is aimed at balancing the entire body, and so it may take longer to produce benefits than other modalities. As acupressure treatment focuses on the entire body, practitioners can detect or see indications of mild irregularities in the body and prevent the accumulation of fatigue and congestion. Acupressure therapy can be used to relieve pain, reduce muscle tension, improve circulation, and promote deep states of relaxation.

In the treatment of the six body types, type T is more fit for acupressure treatment than other groups are. Type P, for instance, has tension and is resistant to exterior pressure or stimulation, and will benefit more with hyperthermal modality prior to acupressure. In certain cases, type P patients are recommended to avoid manual therapy without heat stimulation, as one type P symptom is peripheral vasoconstriction, which is skin and muscle tension that has already developed in the area. Adding more tension or stimulation can cause internal bleeding or muscle contraction. It will be more beneficial to loosen and relax the tension with sufficient heat therapy to dilate peripheral blood vessels before employing manual

therapy. When you go for a spa treatment or massage therapy, the warm shower or hot tub bath before therapy is effective in releasing tension before other stimulation.

HOME SETTING

Half-Body Bath

Hydrotherapy is a well-known, cost-effective remedy in both Eastern and Western cultures. It has been developed as one of the traditional Chinese medicine treatment methods, which can be applied for detoxifying, pain relief, weight control, and clarifying the skin, depending on the characteristics of the diseases. There are three important components of therapeutic bath remedies: (1) the herbal formulation that can be prescribed, depending on the condition; (2) the water temperature and duration (time and frequency); and (3) the applied location, that is, whole-body immersion, half-body bath, foot bath, hand bath, eye bath, and so forth.

Before prescribing an herbal bath formula, practitioners will ask questions and diagnose the symptoms and signs in accordance with traditional medicine criteria prior to establishing a treatment plan. This will show the terms as used in TCM: upper Jiao, middle Jiao, lower Jiao, deficiency, excess, and stagnation. These terms include the common conditions, such as edema, myalgia, dermatitis, and venous insufficiency.

A bath in itself has enormous effects on our body and spirit, while it calms the mind and relaxes musculoskeletal tension, as well as aids a good night's sleep. Hydrotherapy can be used for either relaxing or stimulating blood circulation and the peripheral and central nervous system.

Benefits of Herbal Bath Treatments

- Promote blood circulation
- Alleviate transudate edema
- Facilitate cardiovascular function
- Excrete metabolic skin waste
- Aid sleep and calm the mind

The best time for a half-body bath is between 7:00 and 9:00 p.m., one to two hours prior to bedtime. The water should be a little warmer than normal body temperature 98.6°F–102.2°F (97°F–99°F). Before soaking your body, test the temperature of the water with your hands. In a half-body bath, only soak below the umbilicus; your upper body should be dry. At first, it takes longer for forehead perspiration to break out. It will take 20 minutes or more to begin sweating.

If you have severe venous congestion or vein problems, you should ask your health practitioner before embarking on hydro-therapy. This therapeutic bath is a medicinal remedy and needs preconsultation with a practitioner.

Scrub and Moxa Soap

While treating patients for body reshaping, bathing and showering are recommended as extended home treatment modalities. It is recommended that you examine your body for any abnormalities while taking your daily bath or shower. By bathing and showering regularly, you improve your skin's hygiene and the blood circulation of your lower extremities. Skin is shed daily, as new cells grow and reach the surface every one to two months. The rate of skin cell turnover actually slows down as we age due to changes in hormones and peripheral blood circulation. Using scrub products helps to exfoliate the shedding of superficial dead skin cells and stimulates blood flow.

The benefits of body scrubs are

- Exfoliation can help to slough off dead skin.
- They increase blood flow to the skin surface.
- A rubbing and mild pressing action can help move and drain lymphatic systems.
- They refresh the skin's texture.

For boosting the effectiveness of treatment, moxa soap is recommended for certain conditions, such as scar tissue, severe lymphatic congestion, skin trouble, and blood circulation problems. For treatment of types T and S, I have started to make moxa soap for patients. Moxa soap is made of one-year-fermented moxa floss in special fluids.

Muscle Meridian Stretching

The muscle meridian system has been developed as the part of physical therapy in China for maintaining body posture and as a health exercise. Qi gong is a holistic system of motion and postural coordination with proper breathing and connecting of the inner organ systems. Traditionally, Qi gong practices aim to cultivate health, train spirituality, and balance Qi, especially in martial art. In my clinic, the basic concepts of muscle meridian movement are reported after treatment.

Connect Your Inner Motions

Even though we are not aware of it, our inner body system is constantly moving. In fact, if you feel internal motions such as palpitations or shortness of breath, these are possibly irregular symptoms and signs of ailment. Nevertheless, if you connect your inner body motion, you easily reach meditation moments.

Find your pulse on your wrist with your fingertips, and then wait for a while; you will feel the definite rhythmic beats from your wrist pulse. While you put your fingertips on your wrist, focus your breathing and the beat of your pulse. These two essential body beats are different, and if you focus on them one by one, you can feel the two different rhythms at the same time. Most of the time, we are focused on our outer environment and ignore our body. This newfound awareness will be a good start to maintaining your health.

Practice Moving Your Hands and Feet Slowly and Gently

Just as your life has a direction, most motion and movement have the intention of acting "toward," which is a directional characteristic. Once the direction is decided upon, then the motion is followed, and most directing motion is initiated by the distal body, such as the fingers and toes.

First, loosen your arms and focus on not locking your joints; then try to move your second finger toward the right and left in a circular motion. Then decide on one direction that your finger will follow and move your arm gently in the same direction while focusing on your second finger.

The distal segment can be influenced by proximal segment motion, especially soft small movements. If we need more powerful motions and movements, our joints lock and tense up to resist external shocks. Even posture that is maintained for long periods will result in locking

the joints and maintaining a bending posture. Pressing the joints together causes increased stability, while traction facilitates movement. For loosening the extremities, unlock all joints and start to move your fingers and toes with intentional directional motion.

During physical rehabilitation, dynamic muscle motion can also be emphasized on distal movements. Distal movements, such as finger and toe movements, should occur first and should be completed no later than halfway through the motion pattern to proximal muscles and joints.

Circular Motions

Muscle meridians cover the entire body in the relationship of yin and yang. However, on the extremities, three yin and three yang meridians flow on the six dimensional aspects that are connected to neighboring meridians. On the torso area, three yang feet meridians cover the front, back, and side.

Unlike movements of flexion and extension of joints, a muscle meridian balance test can be done by the circular movements of several joints, such as ankles, wrists, arms, legs, and the neck and waist area. The circular motions are continuous movements turning side to side. This motion is important to diagnose and treat body reshaping of the six body types.

For waist circular motion, initial practice and stretching with a pillow are recommended for type M2, because sudden movement can cause muscle tightness and can be rather uncomfortable.

Pillow stretching includes lying down with a pillow under your midback area, side of body, or abdomen, depending on your position. Once you feel the waist and back area loosen, twisting your waist is an exercise good for strengthening your oblique muscles and the side muscles of your abdomen.

These three steps in muscle meridian stretching methods are recommended for each body type's treatment session.

Diet and Nutrition

Diet Recommendations

Asian food recipes and varieties are countless and include a huge variety of different cooking styles, food sources, and dietary references. Even though it may be difficult to identify the most common main food due to regional varieties, the basic philosophy of cooking and selecting food depends on understanding food quality and its characteristics.

Each food relates to an element of internal organ function, and food classification follows the four basic energetic criteria, such as flavor, thermal nature, organ network, and direction of movement. Similar to Chinese herbal mixtures, certain food combinations are prescribed because of their specific functions, tastes, and Qi properties. For example, if someone has common cold symptoms, they will be told to cook with spicy ingredients, such as green onion or ginger, to induce sweating and promote the relief of symptoms. Eastern diets have developed through empirical observations and are used to treat medical conditions.

When selecting foods, it is beneficial to consider the body condition, the weather, and the individual's emotions. Proper portions and the right choice of food can benefit your body, which has a medicinal effect on body function. If you choose the wrong foods, it can be harmful to your health.

Sleep and Breakfast Habit

I sometimes recommend that my patients skip dinner or eat before 6:00 p.m. during body-reshaping treatment periods. This is because several types and conditions need a 12-hour fasting period in order to gain good results from treatment sessions. Sleep takes up most of the fasting period and breakfast is the break of fasting, which alerts and fuels brain function.

If you eat a late dinner or overeat at dinnertime, it may lead to a restless sleep because when we sleep, our digestive system slows down and becomes sluggish. Furthermore, salivary flow is reduced during sleep, causing a dry mouth in the morning. During sleep, all the muscles relax except those of the diaphragm. The relaxation of the sphincters between the intestinal sections helps to prepare for excretion soon after you wake up and your intestine is active.

For this reason, eating late at night is not recommended, as our inactive state will prevent enzymes and stomach acids from converting food to energy. This causes a bloated feeling during the day. Bloating and congestion are not good, especially for the type P group. The 12-hour fasting diet is usually recommended for instituting daily healthy eating habits.

It is well known that skipping breakfast is associated with a larger waist circumference, metabolic risk factors, and unhealthy lifestyle behaviors. One study suggests that eating in the morning is more satiating and may reduce the total energy intake throughout the day. Busy mornings make it hard to prepare a good solid meal and to even have 30 minutes to enjoy breakfast in your dining room. Instead of warm solid meals, more and more people choose simple juice protein, soft cereal, or liquids to feed their empty stomachs. Hunger suppression and the sensation of fullness depend on the volume of ingested food rather than calories consumed. Moreover, gastrointestinal activity is distinctly different, depending on whether liquids or solid foods are ingested.

Most healthy individuals usually stop eating when they feel full enough. This mechanism is related to the physical stretch on stomach walls induced by the volume of food ingested. According to a TCM author, the stomach's main function is that of "rotting and ripening" food. Before propulsion into the small intestine, ingested food is prepared for digestion and absorption in the stomach. This initial stage of digestion takes several hours to break down and reduce the size of solid meal components.

This process involves fundic relaxation and contraction, the proximal part of the stomach associated with early satiety. The gastric emptying duration is about 240 minutes for solid food. For this reason, if you eat solid food for breakfast and lunch, you can reduce the extra caloric snack or sweet drink between mealtimes.

Personal Planning

It is important to set a realistic goal on the steps of your life ladder. Small achievements can lead to continued motivation. Maintaining a healthy lifestyle does not have a due date, nor is it a quick fix. Your plan should aim at forming basic practical habits throughout your lifetime.

You can lose weight in several months or weeks if you remain dedicated. And you can take a flattering picture by exaggerating your posture. However, these feelings of accomplishment do not indicate a condition of good health.

Your body is constantly changing, day and night, bloating and depressed, taller and shorter, and swelling and wrinkling. We do not live for a one-day photo shoot or a big event. Well-being is the fundamental purpose, and weight loss or body reshaping is the intentional direction to that purpose.

The methods for attaining health are in your lifetime and lifestyle, and cannot be obtained by the number on the scale or the picture in your imagination. Here are some tips for personal planning:

- Set one habit goal each season—four healthy habits per year. Formation of habits takes time, at least three months, so establish a few healthy habits and try them one by one each seasonal quarter.
- Start with distal motions and continue with medial movements and exercises. Sudden movement or exercise of large muscle groups can lead to muscle tenderness or injury; therefore, body performance must have a good sense of dynamics controlled by individual muscle and tendon movements. Before starting an exercise program, soften and loosen your distal extremities at home regularly.
- Check your whole body, morning and night. In the morning, scrubbing the skin can help to awaken your body, so spend more time scrubbing your arms and legs. At night, a 20-minute bath three times a week is recommended. Otherwise, a 15-minute footbath is recommended. Unlike with morning

scrubs, it is a good idea to focus on the tendon and sole of the foot.

- Food and basic meal philosophies are harmonizing, not discriminating. Prior to establishing a diet plan, your gut system and circulatory system should be checked. A healthy digestive system based on a relaxed state is more important than your food selection.

9

Specific Clinical Cautions and Application

MUSCLE MERIDIAN ACUPUNCTURE NEEDLING

I have rarely seen adverse effects from acupuncture treatments. However, several people have shown some signs of discomfort following treatment.

Needle Pinpoint Allergic Reaction

This condition occurs during the treatment session and immediately after needling. Patients did not complain or notice, but a small area surrounding the needlepoint turned red and became swollen. The red swelling usually disappeared within an hour or two. Type P patients have this condition more than other types. To prevent this condition, the hyperthermal method is to be used at the same time or prior to acupuncture needling. After treatment, a half-body bath is recommended with moxa soap at home.

Sore Muscles and a Heavy Feeling after Needling

Since the muscle meridian acupuncture technique focuses on the eccentric and concentric muscles and surrounding tissue, muscle aches are to be expected. The eccentric muscle area, especially, will be sensitive and swollen for two to three days after treatment.

This pain is similar to postexercise pain and may be accompanied by a warm sensation within the muscles.

Bruising

A bruise may be present one or two days after treatment in stretched muscle areas. The most common areas for bruising to occur are at the back of the arm, on the back, and on the upper chest, at the midline of the abdomen. The bruising is not from a direct puncture of the vein, but is due to leakage from the blood vessels in the eccentric contracted muscle. In my clinical

155

experiences, if bruising shows one to two days after needling, the healing process is faster than when there is no bruising present.

Tiredness, Fatigue, and Sleep

Type P patients are more likely to report fatigue after muscle meridian treatment. Usually, type P tension patients live in a state of tension and stress and struggle to rest and relax. The body is then adapted to the extreme levels of continued strain, so the relaxed muscle or feeling of relaxation is seen as a sign of sickness, weakness, or fatigue. Nevertheless, they also mention that their sleep pattern is much improved after treatments.

GASTROINTESTINAL RESUSCITATION AND MOXA TREATMENT

Loose Stool and Gurgling Sound

During the gastrointestinal resuscitation (GIR) treatment with a moxa pad, patients feel relaxed and experience a loosening of the tension almost immediately. However, patients report a change in bowel movement on the night of the treatment session or the next day. It is usually a loose stool without any foul odor, or possibly an isolated incident of diarrhea symptoms accompanied by gurgling sounds. After the bowel movement, the abdominal area feels looser and patients report subjective emotional stability.

Hypochondriac Itchiness

Type M patients are treated with moxa oil instead of smoked moxa during GIR sessions. While treating the skin attached to the hypochondriac muscle, some patients have experienced isolated allergic reactions, such as redness, skin swelling, and itchiness. Most symptoms are gone within three to five days without any medication. A half-body bath can help reduce symptoms. This case often occurs in the area of protruding sixth, seventh, eighth, and ninth ribs, where congested lymphatic fatty tissues are present.

Bloating and Nausea

Several type M3 and type S patients have reported bloating of the abdomen and nausea after GIR treatment sessions. This is more likely to happen when patients are treated several times using the same methods. Smoked moxa is usually very hot on the abdomen, but these individuals do not feel the sensation of heat during several of the sessions. However, when they start feeling the skin sensations, they also become bloated and nauseous. Should this discomfort occur, the treatment method is alternated and adjusted more often. It is relieved after several GIR sessions.

MOXA OIL AND GUA SHA

Bruising

After applying moxa oil on the skin and scraping, a bruise may cover a wide area. It becomes visible within a day or two following treatment and fades two or three days later. In type M3 patients, the inner thigh is the common area for bruising to occur, and in type M1 patients, the medial side of the arm is a common site. This bruise condition occurs in most type M3 patients. The patient experiences a hot or warm feeling on the skin immediately following treatment.

Allergic Reaction

Moxa oil rarely results in an allergic reaction on the skin. However, it may occur in individuals who suffer from atopic dermatitis that is suppressed with medication.

The allergic reaction may occur when muscle weakness and atrophy are present in the problem area. In this case, muscle meridian therapy is needed.

CUPPING

Petechia

Cupping on areas of peripheral blood congestion often displays a spotted, bleeding reaction under the skin known as petechia. It is commonly found in an eccentric contracted muscle area with chronic swelling or congestion. The petechia disappears within three to five days of treatment. The red spots turn dark purple and yellow color before fading.

Appendix: Facial Rejuvenation from Asian Wisdom

Face diagnosis is an important part of the observation in traditional Chinese medicine (TCM). The human body is an inseparable whole, and the face is like a mirror, reflecting physiological function and pathological changes in TCM. The pathological changes of zang-fu (organs and viscera) can be directly diagnosed by inspecting changes in complexion and eye expression.

According to the *Huang Di Nei Jing*, an ancient Chinese medical text treated as the fundamental doctrinal source, Ling Shu, the Qi, and blood of the 12 primary channels and the 365 network vessels ascend to the face. This emphasizes the importance of the complexion as an indication of the general state of health.

Facial cosmetic acupuncture and rejuvenation treatment were performed exclusively for emperors' wives and mistresses, for nobility, and for the wealthy in Eastern countries for thousands of years. The written record was handed down from the Sun dynasty from more than 800 years ago. In Korea, acupuncture meridian massage is, even now, one of the most popular methods for antiaging and promoting blood circulation on the face.

The facial balance acupuncture protocol delivers great success, as shown by before and after clinical records. Facial balance acupuncture utilizes a combination of modalities, including acupuncture, herbal formula, gua sha, and heating methods, for helping the outer appearance, as well as inner health. Before applying these treatments, the practitioner diagnoses underlying causes of imbalance and works to correct the root cause. TCM diagnostic techniques include pulse monitoring, tongue observation, face examination, and taking a history for identifying and treating the major organ imbalances in the body that cause aging and skin imperfections (wrinkles and fine lines appear when there are imbalances in the body). Facial balance acupuncture treats the appearance as well as the inner beauty, body, and mind.

POSTURE AND FACE CONDITIONS

Type M1: Easily swollen, especially after poor sleep. This condition is from diaphragmatic breathing problems. The initial swelling symptoms possibly develop to become a flabby chin and ears, and wrinkles around the eyes.

Type M2: Acne or skin discoloration on the face. Chronic sinusitis results in swollen cheeks and enlarged pores. The straight wrinkle between eyebrows is a common symptom.

Type M3: Overall dark complexion and eyelids indicate an allergic reaction. Swollen eye area and forehead wrinkles are common symptoms.

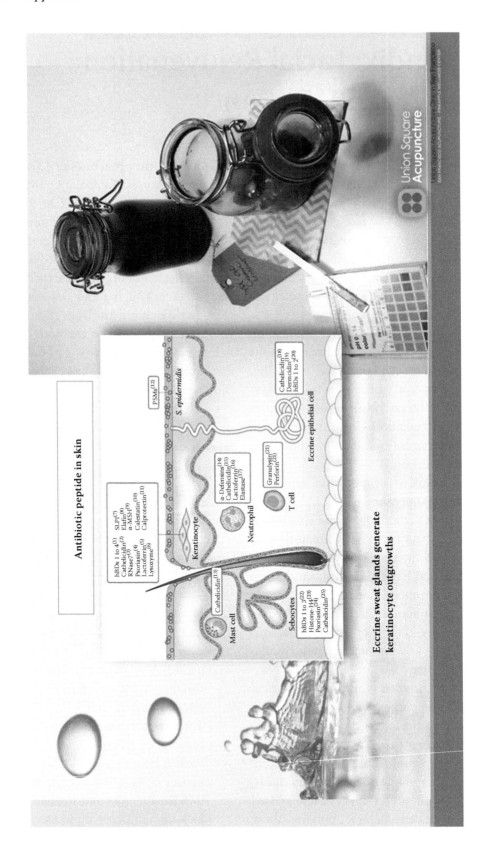

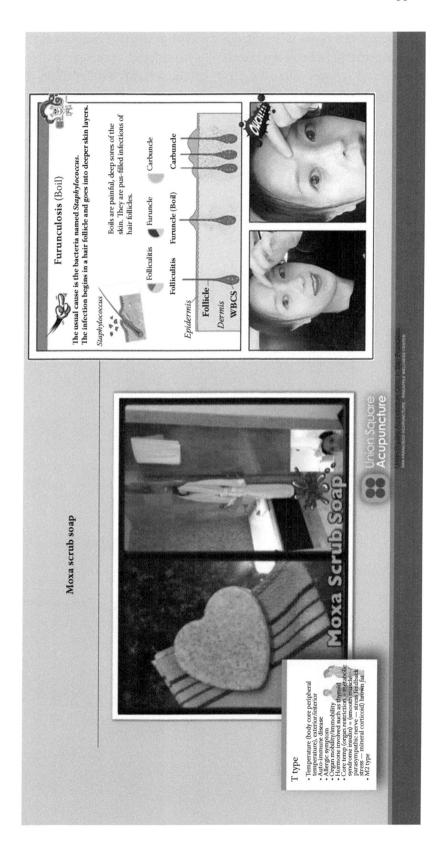

162 • Appendix

Type P: There are two types of wrinkles that indicate whether a body is relaxed or in a state of tension. The straight wrinkles indicate tension in the internal body condition. Facial skin tension indicates a stressed condition, mostly of the breathing system.

Type T: Internal heat or cold is visible in the facial complexion color and the quality of skin, such as dry or wet. Internal cold is presented as a pale complexion and thick skin, whereas internal heat is shown by a dark color and dry skin quality.

Index

This index includes the appendix. Page numbers with "f" and "n" refer to figures and footnotes, respectively.

艾 (Ai Ye), 147
五行 (Five phasic cycle), 37
张仲景 (Zhang Zhong, Jing), 39, 44

A

Abdominal cavity, 17
Abdominal distension, 103, 129
Abdominal muscles, 102, 131
Abdominal obesity, 34, 100
Abdominal pain, 25, 113
Abdominal peritoneum, 25
Abdominal scars, 25
Abductor digiti minimi muscle, 142
Achilles tendon, 4, 109, 111
Acne, 62
Acupressure, 148–149
Acupuncture
    acupuncture meridian, 13–14, 143–144, 155–156
    bruxism and, 32
    goal, 122, 123
    obesity and, 34
    peripheral neuropathies and, 29
    scars and, 28
    significance, 20
Acupuncture and Moxibustion, 146
Acupuncture meridian, 13–14, 143–144, 155–156
Adductor brevis muscle, 136
Adductor longus muscle, 134, 135, 136
Adductor magnus muscle, 136
Adductor minimus muscle, 136
ADH, *see* Antidiuretic hormone (ADH)
Adhesion-related disorders (ARD), 25–26, 113, 114
Adrenal medulla, 42
Aggression (anger)
    digestive system and, 11, 33
    internal organs and, 32
    tension headaches, 67
    three foot yang meridians and, 132
    type S body, 78
Aging, 7, 39, 49, 102
Air Qi, 15
Ai Ye (艾), 147
Alcohol
    body fluids, 43
    bruxism, 32

digestive system, 11
peripheral neuropathies, 29
tension headache, 67
type P body, 62, 93
type S body, 79
Aldosterone, 42
Alkali ingestion, 47
Allergic response, 7, 157
Allergy
    allergic reactions
        cells responsible, 7
        GIR and moxa treatment, 156
        homeostasis, 33
        moxa oil and gua sha, 157
        needle pinpoint, 155
        obesity, 18
        type M2 body, 100
        type M3 body, 159
        type T body, 71
    medication, 33
    skin allergy, 132, 139, 140
    symptoms, 70
Allostasis, 36
ALS, *see* Amyotrophic lateral sclerosis (ALS)
Amylase, 15
Amyotrophic lateral sclerosis (ALS), 46
Anabolism, 20, 48
Angiogenesis, 7, 27
Angiotensin, 42
Ankles
    equinus, 54–55
    pain
        type M3 body, 113
        type P body, 62
        type S body, 78, 83
        type T body, 71
    significance, 111–112
    toe movement and, 112
    type M2 body, 100
    venous insufficiency and, 73
Ankylosing spondylitis, 134
Anterior longitudinal ligament, 136
Anterior pelvic tilt syndrome, 102
Anterior sacrococcygeal ligament, 136
Antidepressants, 33
Antidiabetic drugs, 33

163

164 • Index

Antidiuretic hormone (ADH), 42, 83
Antihistamines, 33
Antihypertensive agents, 33
Anxiety
  body fluids, 42
  body posture, 30
  depression, 32–33
  digestive system, 11, 26, 33
  exercise, 49
  hypocalcemia, 47
  metabolic acidosis, 46
  spleen, 33
  three foot yang meridians, 132
  type M1 body, 89, 90, 94
  type M2 body, 100, 104
  type P body, 63
Apocrine sweat glands, 8
Aponeuroses, 9, 28
Appendectomy, 25
Apple-body shape, 49
ARD, *see* Adhesion-related disorders (ARD)
Areola, 8
Arginine vasopressin (AVP), 83
Armpit, 8, 23
Arms, 93, 104, 114
Artemisia iwayomogi, 146
Artemisia montana, 145–146
Artemisia princeps, 145
Artemisia vulgaris, 145, 147
Arthritis, 5, 78, 84, 90, 94
Aschoff, Jürgen, 38
Asian medicine, 16, 20; *see also* Traditional Chinese
        medicine (TCM)
Asthma, 46
Atopic dermatitis, 157
Atrophic scars, 27
Auricularis muscle, 127, 133
Autonomic nervous system (ANS)
    divisions, 63
    imbalance, 71, 79
    peripheral neuropathies, 29
    spleen function and, 14–15
    stress, 65, 137
AVP, *see* Arginine vasopressin (AVP)
Axillae (armpit), 8, 23

B

Back pain
    idiopathic, 148
    lower
        three foot yang meridians, 132
        type M2 body, 99, 102, 103

  type M3 body, 108, 113
  type S body, 78
  postchildbirth complications, 24
  upper, 89, 92, 113, 132
BAT, *see* Brown adipose tissue (BAT)
Beauty, 1, 2, 3
Behavior
    breakfast habit, 152–153; *see also* Eating
    healthy habit and circadian rhythms, 18
    homeostasis, 41, 42
    sleep, 152–153; *see also* Sleep
    type M1, 94
    type M2, 104
    type M3, 114
Belt vessel, 54, 54f
Bernard, Claude, 35
Bicarbonate, 46
Biceps brachii muscle, 129, 130, 142
Biceps femoris muscle, 111, 132
Biological rhythms, 38
Bi syndrome, 83
Bitter taste, 42
Blisters, 8
Bloating
    gastrointestinal resuscitation (GIR) andmoxa
        treatment, 156
    three hand yin meridians, 129
    type M1 body, 89
    type M2 body, 99, 100, 103–104, 105
    type P body, 62
Blood, 122
Blood circulation, 63, 66, 112–113
Blood loss, *see* Hemorrhage
Blood pH homeostasis, 45–46
Blood pressure, in meridian clock cycle, 19f
Blood vessels, 3, 8, 66, 94, 104, 114
BMI (Body mass index), 33–34
Body balance, 110–111
Body cavities, 16–18
Body clock, 3
Body fluids, 16–18, 41–43
Body mass index (BMI), 33–34
Body pH, 46
Body posture
    adhesion-related disorders (ARD), 25
    cellulites and, 9
    congestion and, 5
    emotions and, 29–30
    examination, 4
    face conditions and, 159, 162
    good, 4–5
    homeostasis and, *see* Body posture and
        homeostasis

Index • 165

muscle-tensed posture, 30, 30f
poor, 30
standing posture, 30, 31f
successful health regimens and, 22
Body posture and homeostasis, 35–57
Chinese medicine, balance, and homeostasis,
36–37
eight principles: pattern of body balance
identification, 39–40
homeostasis, 40–43
homeostasis and metabolism, 47–51
immune function and thermoregulation, 43–44
meridians of the body, 51–57
Chong, 52–54, 53f
Dai, 54, 54f
Du, 52, 52f
overview, 51
Ren, 52, 52f
Yang heel, 54–55, 55f
Yang linking, 55–57, 56f
Yin heel, 54–55, 55f
Yin linking, 55–57, 56f
overview, 35–36
traditional Chinese medicine life cycles, 37–39
biological rhythms, 38
kidney and kidney essence, 38–39
overview, 37–38
understanding body homeostasis and
metabolism, 47–51
Wu Xing, 37
Body reshaping
balancing and reshaping your body, 3–4
beauty definition, 6–7
body posture, 4, 5
food, fitness, and fat, 10–11
having healthy body shape, 4–6
learning from man's best friend, 2–3
losing weight, 12
perfect 10 body, 1–2
resetting your digestive system, 11
skin and thermoregulation, 7–8
subcutaneous fat, 8–10
successful health regimens and, 22–23
treatment, 14
Body shapes, 3, 4–6, 11, 14
Body temperature, 19f, 43, 137; see also Skin;
Thermoregulation
Body types
background, 59–60
branches and root, 60
characteristics, 61–62
criteria, 60–61
extraordinary meridians and, 51

illustration, 61f
muscle meridians and, 122–123
skin and, 137–138
type M1 body, 89–98
associated disorders, 94
case study, 94–98
clinical syndrome, 90
criteria, 61
home therapy and caution, 94
illustrative examples, 61f, 90f
mechanism, 90–92, 91f
muscle connection and function, 93
neck wrinkle, 91f
pain, 92–93
postural characteristics, 93–94
quick tips, 89
related condition, 89–90
type P body and, 63, 67, 90, 93
yang, 90, 92, 139f
yin, 90, 92, 93
type M2 body, 98–107
adhesions and, 26
associated disorders, 104
body posture and face conditions, 159
case study, 106–107
clinical syndrome, 99–100
criteria, 61
home care and precautions, 105–106
illustrative examples, 61f, 98f
mechanism, 100–101, 101f, 103f
muscle connections and functions,
101–103
pain, 103–104
postural characteristics, 104
quick tips, 98–99
treatment, 104–105
type M3 body, 107–119
associated disorders, 114
blood circulation, 113
case study, 116–119
clinical syndrome, 108–110
criteria, 61
home therapy and precautions, 115
illustrative examples, 61f
mechanism, 110–111, 110f
muscle sequential connection and function,
111–112
neck wrinkle, 91f
pain, 113–114
postural characteristics, 114
quick tips, 107–108
related condition, 108
treatment, 114–115

166 • Index

type P body, 62–70
    acupressure and, 149
    associated disorders, 67
    case study, 68–70
    clinical syndrome, 63–65
    criteria, 61
    dampness pattern, 18
    definition, 65, 65f
    eating and, 152
    home therapy and caution, 68
    illustrative example, 61f, 62f
    mechanism, 65–66, 65f
    neck wrinkle, 91f
    pain, 66–67, 75
    postural characteristics, 67
    quick tips, 62
    related conditions, 62–63
    treatment, 67–68
    type M1 body and, 63, 67, 90, 93
type S body, 78–87
    associated disorders, 84
    case study, 85–87
    clinical syndrome, 79–82
    criteria, 61
    extraordinary channels and, 39
    home therapy and caution, 85
    illustrative examples, 61f, 78f
    mechanism, 82–83
    pain, 83–84
    postural characteristics, 84
    quick tips, 78
    related conditions, 78–79
    treatment, 84–85
    type P pattern and, 64
type T body, 70–78
    associated disorders, 75
    case study, 76–78
    clinical syndrome, 71–72
    criteria, 61
    dampness pattern, 18
    definition, 71, 71f
    home therapy and caution, 76
    illustrative examples, 61f, 70f
    mechanism, 72–74
    pain, 74–75
    postural characteristics, 75
    quick tips, 70
    related conditions, 70–71
    treatment, 75–76
    type P pattern and, 64
Boils, 161f
Bone, 47, 122
Bone fracture, 5

Bowel movements, 26, 70, 156
Brachioradialis muscle, 129, 130
Breakfast habit, 152–153
Breast, 10, 23
Breech birth, 147
Bronchitis, 46
Brown adipose tissue (BAT), 43
Bruising
    moxa oil and gua sha, 156–157
    muscle meridian acupuncture technique,
        155–156
Bruxism, 32
Buffer systems, 46
Bursitis, 94, 103
Buttocks, 27, 28, 82, 103, 111, 133

C

Caesarian section (C-section), 24–25
Calcium homeostasis, 47
Cannon, Walter, 36
Carbaminohemoglobin, 46
Carbohydrates, 48
Carbon dioxide, 45, 46
Carbonic acid–bicarbonate buffer system, 46
Carbuncle, 161f
Cardiac muscles, 50
Cartilage, 122
Case studies
    type M1 body, 94–98
    type M2 body, 106–107
    type M3 body, 116–119
    type P body, 68–70
    type S body, 85–87
    type T body, 76–78
Catabolism, 48
Cellular homeostasis, 45
Cellulite, 9, 28
Central obesity, 49
Cervical spinal dysfunction, 31
CFS, *see* Chronic fatigue syndrome (CFS)
Channel network, 13; *see also* Meridians
Chinese medicine, 36–37; *see also* Traditional
        Chinese medicine (TCM)
Chinese tui na massage, 20
Chong meridian, 37, 38, 53f
Chronic fatigue syndrome (CFS), 24, 74, 75
Chronic mononucleosis, 75
Circadian rhythms, 3, 18, 19–20, 38
Circulatory system, 38, 48
Cirrhosis, 17
Classic of Difficulties, 51
Clavicle, 94, 104

Climbing muscle, *see* Latissimus dorsi
Clinical cautions and application, 155–157
  cupping, 157
  gastrointestinal resuscitation (GIR) and moxa
    treatment, 156
  moxa oil and gua sha, 156–157
  muscle meridian acupuncture needling, 155–156
Coffee, 42, 43
Cold and hot identification, 40
Cold bi, 83
Cold feet, 62
Cold hands, 62
Cold sensitivity, 70
Cold syndrome, 40
Collagen, 39
Congestions
  abdominal, 9, 16, 18, 100
  back area water, 54
  breathing and circulation, 66
  chest, 124
  definition, 5, 145
  eating, 152
  epigastric, 72
  inner thigh, 124
  intestinal fatty, 130
  joint motion, 83
  lymphatic, 90, 92, 93, 140, 150
  muscle, 23
  pelvic, 114
  sinus, 99, 127
  skin, 141
  type T body, 75
  upper fat, 128
  venous, 145; *see also* Venous insufficiency
Congestive heart failure (CHF), 17
Connective tissue, 7, 17, 121, 122
Constipation, 47, 62, 70, 104, 108, 148
Contracture scars, 27
Convulsions, 145
Coracobrachialis muscle, 93
Core muscles, 54
Corticosteroids, 47
Cortisol, 82
Creatinine, 46
Cupping, 20, 29, 144–145, 157
Cushing syndrome, 84
Cutaneous meridians; *see also* Skin
  body types and, 137–138
  clinical syndrome, 138–141
    Jue yin, 140, 140f
    Shao yang, 139, 139f
    Shao yin, 141, 141f
    Tai yang, 138–139, 138f

  Tai yin, 140, 140f
  Yang ming, 139, 139f
  diagnosis, 137–138
  function of skin, 137
  meridian classification of, 122
  myotome and dermatome, 141–142
  significance, 136–137
  treatment, 138
Cutaneous needle, 138
Cutaneous vasodilation, 7
Cyanosis, 145

D

Dai meridian, 54, 54f
Damp bi, 83
Damp cold, 14
Damp heat, 14
Damp-heat pattern, 18
Dampness, 15, 17, 72, 145, 146
Dangun Wanggeom legend, 146
Dehydration, 41, 43
Deltoid muscle, 101, 128, 142
Depression
  anxiety and, 32–33
  body posture, 30
  digestive system, 11, 26
  exercise, 49
  food restriction, 50
  hypercalcemia, 47
  three foot yang meridians, 132
  treatment, 7
  type M1 body, 90
  type M2 body, 100, 104
  type M3 body, 113
  type S body, 78, 83, 84
  type T body, 70
Dermatitis, 149, 157
Dermatomes, 141–142
Dermis, 7, 27, 161f
Diabetes mellitus, 8, 29, 47, 49, 67, 80
Diagnostic points
  foot Jue yin liver meridian flow, 135
  foot Shao yang gallbladder meridian flow, 133
  foot Shao yin kidney meridian flow, 136
  foot Tai yin spleen muscle meridian flow, 134
  foot Yang ming stomach meridian flow, 134
  hand Shao yang san jiao (triple burner) meridian
    flow, 128
  hand Shao yin heart meridian flow, 130
  hand Tai yang small intestine meridian flow, 127
  hand Tai yin lung muscle meridian flow, 129
  hand Yang ming large intestine meridian flow, 128

168 • *Index*

Diagnostic postures
    foot Jue yin liver meridian flow, 135
    foot Shao yang gallbladder meridian flow, 133
    foot Shao yin kidney meridian flow, 136
    foot Tai yang urinary bladder meridian flow, 132
    foot Tai yin spleen muscle meridian flow, 134
    foot Yang ming stomach meridian flow, 134
    hand Jue yin pericardium muscle meridian flow, 129–130
    hand Shao yang san jiao (triple burner) meridian flow, 128
    hand Shao yin heart meridian flow, 130
    hand Tai yang small intestine meridian flow, 127
    hand Tai yin lung muscle meridian flow, 129
    hand Yang ming large intestine meridian flow, 128
Diaphragm, 3, 5, 16, 102, 130, 131f
Diaphragm sprain, 130
Diet and nutrition, 3, 18, 20, 21, 152–153
Digestive system, 11, 29, 48
Diuretics, 84
Diurnal rhythms, 38
Divergent meridians, 122
Dizziness, 62, 78, 114
Dogs, 2–3
Dopaminergic system disturbances, 32
Dorsal interossei muscle, 142
Drug use, 32
Dry eyes, 62
Dry-heat pattern, 18
Dry mouth, 62
Dry skin, 62
Du14, 52, 52f
Du meridian, 52, 52f
Dynamic motion, 36
Dyslipidemia, 49
Dyspepsia, 26, 104

E

Earache, 89, 127
Ear canal, 8
Eating, *see* Diet and nutrition
Eccrine sweat glands, 7, 43, 160f
Edema
    disorders, and dampness, 17
    exudate, 17
    lipedema, 82–83
    pulmonary, 46
    renal failure, 51
    spleen, 73
    transudate, 17
    treatment, 144–145, 149
    venous insufficiency, 112

Eight-principle pattern, 39–40
Elbows, 28
Emotions, 11, 29–30, 32–33; *see also specific emotions*
Emphysema, 46
Endocrine system, 48, 50; *see also* Homeostasis
Endometriosis, 25
ENS, *see* Enteric nervous system (ENS)
Enteric nervous system (ENS), 3, 11
Epicarnius muscle, 133
Epidermis, 6–7, 27, 161f
Epigastric pain, 26
Epinephrine, 42
Epithelial tissue, 121
Epsom salts, 65
Equinus, 54–55
Erector spinae muscle, 99, 111, 115
Estrogen, 47, 83
Exercise
    effects
    benefits, 46, 49–50
        lymphatic fluids, 72, 73
        respiration, 45
        skeletal muscle, 64, 65, 66
        skin, 9, 66
        vacuity pattern, 40
    as healthy habit, 18
    as stress, 65
    sweating, 8, 41
Extensor carpi radialis longus, 128, 142
Extensor carpi radialis brevis, 142
Extensor digitorum longus muscle, 109, 128, 133, 134, 142
Extensor hallucis longus muscle, 109, 135, 136, 142
Exterior syndrome, 39
Exterior versus interior identification, 39–40
External oblique muscle, 102, 131
Extraordinary meridians, 39, 51, 122
Extremities
    adhesion-related disorders (ARD), 26
    pain and digestion, 27
    peripheral nervous system damage, 29
    spleen function in TCM, 15–16
    type P body, 63–64
Exudate edema, 17
Eyelids, 8
Eyer, Joseph, 36

F

Face, 26, 93, 104, 114
Face diagnosis, 159
Facial rejuvenation, 159–162

Facial swelling, 71
Falciform ligament, 135
Fat; *see also* Obesity; *specific body types*
    body motion, 8
    body shape, 3
    calcium, 47
    distribution, 114
    food, fitness, and, 10–11
    muscles and, 9
    subcutaneous, 8–10, 23–24
    thermoregulation, 7–8, 43–44
    visceral fat, 8–9
Fatigue
    chronic, 24, 74, 75
    muscle meridian acupuncture, 156
    respiratory acidosis, 46
    type M1 body, 89
    type M2 body, 99
    type T body, 70
Fear, 11, 33
Feet
    eccrine sweat glands, 7
    flat, 80, 102
    muscle meridian stretching, 151
    traditional Chinese medicine (TCM), 112
    type M2 body, 103, 104, 109
    type P body, 62, 65
Femur, 111
Fever, 43–44, 145
FGID, *see* Functional gastrointestinal disorders
    (FGID)
Fibroblasts, 7, 27
Fibromyalgia, 7, 74, 75, 108, 114
Fibrous connective tissue, 122
Fiburalis longus muscle, 133
Fingers
    dermatomes, 141
    muscle meridians, 123, 126
    type M1 body, 94
    type M2 body, 104
    type M3 body, 114
    type T body, 71
Fire cupping, 144
Five phasic cycle (五行), 37
Flat-back posture, 109
Flexor carpi ulnaris muscle, 127
Flexor digitorum brevis muscle, 136
Flexor digitorum profundus muscle, 130, 142
Flexor digitorum superficialis muscle, 142
Folliculitis, 161
Food, 8, 10–11, 42, 98; *see also* Diet and nutrition
Food intolerance, 70
Foot Jue yin liver meridian flow, 135, 135f
Foot pain, 108, 112, 132

Foot Shao yang gallbladder meridian flow, 133, 133f
Foot Shao yin kidney meridian flow, 135–136, 136f
Foot Tai yang urinary bladder meridian flow,
    132–133, 132f
Foot Tai yin spleen muscle meridian flow, 134–135,
    135f
Foot Yang ming stomach meridian flow, 133–134, 134f
Frontal headache, 99
Frustration, 78
Function versus structure, 50–51
Functional dyspepsia, 26, 104
Functional gastrointestinal disorders (FGID),
    26–27, 103, 104
Fu organs, 51
Furuncle, 161f
Furunculosis, 161f

G

Gallbladder, 18, 19f, 20, 51
Gastrectomy, 47
Gastrocnemius muscle, 109, 111, 112, 132
Gastrointestinal malabsorption, 17
Gastrointestinal resuscitation (GIR), 26, 105,
    147–148, 156
GIR, *see* Gastrointestinal resuscitation (GIR)
Gluteus maximus muscle, 103, 111, 133
Gluteus medius muscle, 27, 103, 133
Gonadal steroids, 82
Gout, 84
Gracilis muscle, 135
Granulation, 7
Green tea, 42–43
Gua sha, 7, 20, 29, 145–146, 156–157
Gustatory nerve, 31

H

Habits, 18, 21, 152–153; *see also* Lifestyle and
    homeostasis
Hair follicles, 10, 160f
Hair loss, 8, 63, 90
Half-body bath, 149–150, 155, 156
Hamstrings muscle, 103, 111
Hand Jue yin pericardium muscle meridian flow,
    129–130, 129f
Hands
    eccrine sweat glands, 7
    muscle meridian stretching, 151
    muscle meridians, 123, 126
    type M1 body, 94
    type M2 body, 104
    type M3 body, 114
    type P body, 62

170 • Index

Hand Shao yang san jiao (triple burner) meridian
    flow, 127–128, 128f
Hand Shao yin heart meridian flow, 130, 130f
Hand Tai yang small intestine meridian flow, 127, 127f
Hand Tai yin lung muscle meridian flow, 129, 129f
Hand Yang ming large intestine meridian flow, 128,
    128f
Hand Yin muscle meridian reference, 130–132
Headache
    frontal, 99
    heat exhaustion, 43
    migraine, 94
    occipital, 108, 134
    tension, 62, 66–67
Health, 14, 98
Heart
    congestion, 145
    emotions, 32
    exercise, 66
    homeostasis, 50
    in meridian clock cycle, 19, 19f
    obesity, 33
    taste and, 42
    type M3 and blood circulation, 112
    upper jiao, 17
    Zang organs, 51
Heartburn, 99
Heat, 8
Heat bi, 83
Heat exhaustion, 43
Heat injury, 43
Heat intolerance, 29
Heat stone room sauna (zzim jil bang), 147
Heatstroke, 43
Heat syndrome, 40
Hematoma, 145
Hemoglobin, 46
Hemophilia, 145
Hemorrhage, 41
Hemorrhoids, 62
Heparin, 7
Hepatic disorders, 17, 104
Hernia, 62
Hip bursitis, 103
Hip extensors, 99
Hip flexors, 99, 101, 103
Hip pain, 102, 103, 108, 114
Histamine, 7
Homeostasis, 40–43
    Chinese medicine, and balance, 36–37
    definition, 8
    dysfunction, 41
    extraordinary blood vessels and, 57
    lifestyle and, 49–50

metabolism and, 47–51
    origin, 36
    structure versus function, 50–51
Horary clock cycle, 19, 19f
Hot and cold identification, 40
Hot flashes, 147
Huang Di Nei Jing, 159
Hydrostatic pressure, 41
Hydrotherapy, 149
Hyoglossus muscle, 128
Hypercalcemia, 47
Hyperemia, 145
Hyperglycemia, 49
Hyperlipidemia, 84
Hyperpigmentation, 73
Hypertension, 49, 63, 67, 80, 84
Hyperthermal treatment methods, 138, 155
Hyperthermia, 43
Hyperthyroidism, 49, 67, 79, 84
Hypertrophic scars, 27
Hypervolemia, 41
Hypocalcemia, 47
Hypochondriac itchiness, 156
Hypothalamus, 7, 43, 79
Hypothyroidism, 17, 49, 79, 84
Hypovolemia, 41
Hysterectomy, 25

I

IBS (Irritable bowel syndrome), 25, 26, 75, 104
Iliacus muscle, 101
Iliocostalis lumborum muscle, 99, 102, 111
Iliopsoas muscle, 101, 142
Immunization and thermoregulation, 43, 44
Indigestion, 99
Infections, 8, 29, 71
Infertility, 78, 84, 108
Inflammation, 27, 29, 44, 71
Infradian rhythms, 38
Infrared heat, 138
Infraspinatus muscle, 127
Inguinal ligament, 135
Innate immune system, 44
Insomnia, 20, 40
Insulin-like growth factor, 82
Insulin resistance, 49, 84
Intercostal muscles, 17, 129, 130
Intercourse, 25, 40
Interior syndrome, 39–40
Internal cold, 162
Internal heat, 162
Internal oblique muscle, 102, 131
Internal respiratory system, 45

Interstitial cystitis, 25, 75
Intestinal malabsorption syndrome, 47
Intravenous fluids, 41
Irregular menstruation, 78
Irritable bowel syndrome (IBS), 25, 26, 75, 104

J

Ja-Hun, 147
Jet lag, 20
Jing, 122n
Joint pain
    leg, 112
    mechanical, 83
    metabolic, 46, 84
    type M1 body, 90
    type T body, 71
Joy, 32
Jue yin meridian, 19, 140, 140f

K

Keloid scars, 27
Keratinocytes, 160f
Kidney Qi, 39
Kidneys
    emotions and, 33
    extraordinary vessels and, 51
    hydration and, 41
    in meridian clock cycle, 19, 19f
    kidney essence and, 38–39
    kidney Qi, 39
    overhydration, 41
    role, 41–42
    roles, 41, 46, 102
    taste and, 42
    upper jiao, 18
    Zang organs, 51
Kinesiology, 20
Knees
    contracture, 29
    pain
        obese and overweight, 29
        three foot yang meridians, 132
        type M2 body, 99, 102, 103
        type M3 body, 108, 113
        type S body, 83
Kyphosis, 102, 104, 109, 114, 127

L

Lactic acid, 46
Laparoscopy, 25
Large intestine, 18, 19, 19f, 51

Latissimus dorsi muscle
    accessory breathing muscles, 131, 132
    congestion, 23
    shoulder adductor, 93
    three foot yang meridians, 133, 134
    type M2 body, 99, 101–102
Legs
    gastrointestinal resuscitation (GIR), 148
    lipedema, 78, 82–83
    O shape, 81
    traditional Chinese medicine (TCM), 112
    type M2 body, 104
    type M3 body, 108, 114
    venous insufficiency, 73
    X shape, 80
Levator ani muscle, 136
Levatores costarum muscle, 130, 131
Levator scapular muscle, 93, 127, 128
Lifestyle and homeostasis, 49–50; see also Habits
Ligaments, 5, 29, 101, 135, 136
Light sensitivity, 63
Ling Shu, 159
Lipedema, 78, 82–83
Lipids, 48
Lipodermatosclerosis, 73
Lipoma, 4, 102
Liver
    emotions and, 33
    in meridian clock cycle, 19, 19f
    middle Jiao, 18
    taste and, 42
    Zang organs, 51
Longissimus muscle, 102, 111
Longus capitis muscle, 111
Longus coli muscle, 111
Lordosis, 99, 100, 101, 102, 109, 132
Love handles, 80, 99, 102, 132
Lower back, 23–24, 103, 108
Lower erector spinae muscle, 99
Lower Jiao, 18
Lumbosacral fascia, 102
Lumbricals muscle, 142
Lung Qi, 102, 137
Lungs, 51
    emotions and, 32
    lung Qi, 102, 137
    in meridian clock cycle, 19, 19f, 45
    middle Jiao, 17
    osmoregulatory role, 41–42
    roles, 46
    taste and, 42
    Zang organs, 51
Luo-connecting meridians, 122, 122n
Lymphatic congestion, 150

172 • Index

Lymphatic system, 72–73
Lymphedema, 73
Lymphocytes, 44

M

Macrophages, 7
Mai, 79
Malnutrition, 41, 42; *see also* Diet and nutrition
Masseter muscle, 93, 127, 128, 134
Mast cells, 7, 160f
Mastication, 30–31
Medical history, 3, 90
Medulla oblongata, 45
Melatonin, 19f, 20
Menstrual cramping, 62
Meridian clock, 19–20, 19f
Meridians
  basic concept, 45
  classifications, 122
  definition, 13
  extraordinary meridians
    Chong, 52–54, 53f
    Dai, 54, 54f
    Du, 52, 52f
    Ren, 52, 52f
    Yang heel, 54–55, 55f
    Yang linking, 55–57, 56f
    Yin heel, 54–55, 55f
    Yin linking, 55–57, 56f
  muscle, *see* Muscle meridians
  overview, 51
  qi and, 13–14
Metabolic acidosis, 46
Metabolic syndrome, 49, 79, 84
Metabolism, 47–51
  definition, 47–48
  essential organic molecules, 48
  extraordinary blood vessels and, 57
  homeostasis and, 48–49
  lifestyle and homeostasis, 49–50
  pathway in the body, 48
  structure versus function, 50–51
Middle Jiao, 15, 18
Migraine, 94
Milk–alkali syndrome, 47
Ming dynasty, 51
Miraculous Pivot, 45
Moxa
  oil, 145–146, 156–157
  soap, 150
  treatment, 7, 84, 156, 161
Moxibustion, 13, 20, 29, 122, 138, 146–147
Muffin top, *see* Love handles
Mugwort, 145–146

Multifidus, 102, 131f, 133
Muscle meridian acupuncture technique, 143–144,
    155–156
Muscle meridians
  body types and, 122–123
  characteristics, 124–126
    nourishment of muscles, tendons, and skin,
      124–125
    origination from distal body, 126
    pathogenic patterns, 125–126
    three yang and three yin hand and foot
      meridians, 125
  definition, 121–123
  pattern, 124f
  treatments, 126–136
    three foot yang meridians, 132–134
    three foot yin meridians, 134–136
    three hand yang meridians, 127–128
    three hand yin meridians, 128–132
Muscle meridian stretching, 150–152
Muscle meridian therapy, 121–142
  cutaneous meridians, 136–142
  muscle and sinew meridians and cutaneous
    meridians, 121–123
  muscle meridian treatments, 123–136
    characteristics of muscle meridians, 124–126
    muscle meridians, 126–136
Muscles; *see also specific types of muscles*
  body shape, 3
  cardiac, 50, 148
  core muscle, 54
  eye, 26
  nourishment, 124–125
  related in
    foot Jue yin liver meridian flow, 135
    foot Shao yang gallbladder meridian flow, 133
    foot Shao yin kidney meridian flow, 136
    foot Tai yang urinary bladder meridian flow,
      132–133
    foot Tai yin spleen muscle meridian flow, 135
    foot Yang ming stomach meridian flow, 134
    hand Jue yin pericardium muscle meridian
      flow, 130
    hand Shao yang san jiao (triple burner)
      meridian flow, 128
    hand Shao yin heart meridian flow, 130
    hand Tai yang small intestine meridian flow,
      127
    hand Tai yin lung muscle meridian flow, 129
    hand Yang ming large intestine meridian
      flow, 128
  respiratory, 45, 102, 130–132
  skeletal, 50, 65–66, 71, 73, 93, 102, 126
  spleen function in TCM, 15–16
  uterine, 25

Muscles contraction, 5
Muscle tissue, 121
Muscular imbalance, 5
Myalgia, 149
Myofascial pain, 92, 94
Myotome, 141–142

N

Nausea, 46, 47, 72, 156
Neck
    adhesion-related disorders (ARD), 26
    brown fat, 43
    discoloration, 90
    fat, 92
    lymphatic system, 72
    pain
        chronic fatigue syndrome (CFS), 74
        tension headache, 67
        type P body, 62, 63, 64, 67
        type S body, 79
    short, 81
    type M1 body, 93
    type M2 body, 104
    type M3 body, 114
    wrinkle differentiation, 91f
Neck flexors, 111
Needle pinpoint allergic reaction, 155
Negative feedback, 48
Negative-pressure wound therapy (NPWT), 145
Neijing Suwen, 39
Nervous tissue, 121
Neuromuscular disorders, 46
Neutrophils, 44, 160f
NHANES, *see* U.S. National Health and Nutrition
        Examination Survey (NHANES)
Nipples, 8
Norepinephrine, 42
Nose, 8
NPWT, *see* Negative-pressure wound therapy (NPWT)
Numbness, 28, 29
Nutrition, *see* Diet and nutrition
Nutritional Qi, 15

O

Obesity, 33–34
    abdominal, 18, 34, 100
    body imbalances and, 34
    central, 49
    disease and, 33
    hypoventilation syndrome, 46
    metabolic syndromes, 49
    statistics, 33
    steps to, 14

Obesity hypoventilation syndrome, 46
Oblique muscles, 102, 111, 131, 134
Occipital headache, 108, 134
Occlusal discrepancies, 32
Oncotic pressure, 41
Orbicularis oculi muscle, 133
Orbicularis oris muscle, 134
Oromandibular dystonia, 32
Orthostatic intolerance, 75
Osmotic pressure, 41
Osteoporosis, 47, 50
Ovariectomy, 25
Overhydration, 41
Overweight, 14, 29, 33, 49

P

Pain
    abdominal, 25, 113
    back; *see also* Back pain
    digestion and, 27
    epigastric, 26
    hip, 102, 103, 108, 114
    intercourse, 25
    joint pain, *see* Joint pain
    knee, *see* Knees, pain
    myalgia, 149
    myofascial pain, 92, 94
    neck, *see* Neck, pain
    pelvic, 25, 75, 113
    sensation, 92
    shoulder, *see* Shoulder pain
    superficial pain, 92
    toe pain, 108, 112
    type M1 body, 92–93
    type M2 body, 103–104
    type M3 body, 113–114
    type P body, 66–67, 75
    type S body, 83–84
    type T body, 75–76
Palmar interossei muscle, 142
Palms, 7, 64, 124
Palpitations, 46, 57, 62, 151
Panic, 26, 45
Parasympathetic nervous system (PNS), 3, 10, 15
Parotid glands, 31
Paroxysmal extreme pain sensations, 92
Paroxysmal sympathetic hyperactivity, 54
Pathways
    foot Jue yin liver meridian flow, 135
    foot Shao yang gallbladder meridian flow, 133
    foot Shao yin kidney meridian flow, 135
    foot Tai yang urinary bladder meridian flow, 132
    foot Tai yin spleen muscle meridian flow, 134
    foot Yang ming stomach meridian flow, 133

174 • *Index*

hand Jue yin pericardium muscle meridian flow, 129
hand Shao yang san jiao (triple burner) meridian flow, 127
hand Shao yin heart meridian flow, 130
hand Tai yang small intestine meridian flow, 127
hand Tai yin lung muscle meridian flow, 129
hand Yang ming large intestine meridian flow, 128
PCOS, *see* Polycystic ovarian syndrome (PCOS)
Pectoralis major muscle, 93, 129, 131, 134
Pectoralis minor muscle, 93, 129, 131, 134
Pectus carinatum, 129
Pelvic cavity, 17, 28
Pelvic congestion syndrome, 114
Pelvic floor disorder, 114
Pelvic floor muscles, 131f
Pelvic pain, 25, 75, 113
Pelvic peritoneum, 25
Pelvis, 110
Pericardium, 17, 19, 19f
Peripheral nervous system (PNS), 29
Peripheral neuropathies, 28–29
Peripheral vasoconstriction, 149
Peritoneum, 135
Peroneus brevis muscle, 142
Peroneus longus muscle, 142
Personality type, 32
Personal planning, 153–154
Petechiae, 157
pH, 45–46
Phagocytosis, 44
Phleboliths, 114
Phlegm, 29
Phosphate buffer system, 46
Phosphate homeostasis, 47
Pillow stretching, 151–152
Plain Question, 136
Plantar fasciitis, 29
Plum blossom, 29
Pneumonia, 46
PNS (Parasympathetic nervous system), *see* Parasympathetic nervous system (PNS)
PNS (Peripheral nervous system), *see* Peripheral nervous system (PNS)
Polycystic ovarian syndrome (PCOS), 84
Polyphenols, 42
Postpartum depression, 104
Posttraumatic stress disorder (PTSD), 26, 67
Pregnant woman, 145; *see also* Type M2 body
Premenstrual syndrome (PMS), 84
Prenatal Qi, 15
Primary meridians (Jing), 122, 122n
Protein buffer system, 46
Proteins, 48

PTSD, *see* Posttraumatic stress disorder (PTSD)
Pubic symphysis, 102
Pubis, 25
Pulmonary edema, 46
Pulmonary ventilation, 45
Pulse monitoring, 159
Pungent taste, 42
Pyramidalis muscle, 135
Pyrogens, 44

Q

Qi
    kidney, 39, 102
    lung, 102, 137
    meridian system and, 13–14
    nutritional, 15
    stomach, 15
    true, 15
    Wei, 56
Qi gong, 150
Qi level, 39
Quadratus lumborum muscle, 102
Quadriceps femoris muscle, 103, 134, 142
Que, Bian, 146

R

Range of motion, 94, 104, 114
Rapid eye movement (REM), 5
Rashes, 8
Receivers of the treatment, 21–34
    adhesion-related disorders (ARD), 25–26
    body reshaping and successful health regimens, 22–23
    bruxism, 32
    caesarian section (C-section), 24–25
    cellulite, 28
    depression and anxiety, 32–33
    emotional expression by the body, 29–30
    functional gastrointestinal disorders (FGID), 26–27
    major scars, 27–28
    medications history complications, 33
    obesity, 33–34
    peripheral neuropathies, 28–29
    postchildbirth complications, 24
    subcutaneous fat, 23–24
    temporomandibular joint (TMJ), 30–32
    weight loss or diet life versus your life, 21–22
Rectococcygeus muscle, 136
Rectus abdominis muscle, 25, 99, 102, 111, 131, 134
Rectus femoris, 101
Rectus sheath, 25
REM, *see* Rapid eye movement (REM)

Renal failure, 47
Renal insufficiency, 84
Renin, 42
Ren meridian, 37, 38
Repletion and vacuity identification, 40
Repletion pattern, 40
Reproductive problems, 134
Respiration
    abdominal cavity fluid, 99
    autonomic nervous system (ANS), 15
    cellular, 45
    circulation and, 66
    external, 45
    metabolic excretion, 46
    muscle imbalances, 123
    muscles, 45, 102, 130–132
    paroxysmal sympathetic hyperactivity, 54
    traditional Chinese medicine (TCM), 102
    type M1 body, 94
    type M2 body, 99, 100
    type M3 body, 110
Respiratory acidosis, 46
Respiratory homeostatic balance, 44–45
Rhomboids muscles, 127, 131

S

Sadness, 32, 90, 94; *see also* Depression
Saliva, 15, 31
Salivary glands, 31
Salt intake, 41–43
San Jiao (Triple Burner), 17, 18, 19f, 20, 127–128
Scalene muscle, 93, 131
Scapular alata, *see* Winged scapular (scapular alata)
Scar formation, 27
Scars, 27–28, 78, 79, 108, 150
Scleroderma fibroblasts, 7
SCM, *see* Sternocleidomastoid (SCM)
Scoliosis, 109, 114
Scrub and moxa soap, 150
Sea of blood, 52, 53f
Sea of yin, 52, 52f
Second brain, *see* Enteric nervous system (ENS)
Semimembranosus muscle, 111, 135
Semispinalis capitis muscle, 133
Semitendinosus muscle, 111, 132
Sensitivity to touch, 29
Serous fluid, 14–15
Serratus anterior muscle, 93, 129, 130, 131
Serratus posterior inferior muscle, 130, 131, 135
Serratus posterior superior muscle, 130, 131
Shang Han Lun (220 A.D.), 39, 44
Shao yang meridian, 20, 139, 139f
Shao yin meridian, 19, 141, 141f

Shiatsu, 148
Shortness of breath (dyspnea), 46, 62, 80, 94, 129, 131
Shoulder pain
    tension headache, 67
    three hand yang meridians, 127
    type M1 body, 89
    type M2 body, 99, 102
    type M3 body, 113
    type P body, 62
    type S body, 79
Sinew therapy, *see* Muscle meridians
Sinusitis, 17, 89, 127
Sitting, 9, 99, 100, 130
Skeletal muscles, 50, 65–66, 71, 73, 93, 102, 126
Skin
    allergy, 132, 139, 140
    body shape and, 3
    body types and, 137–138
    cold exposure, 44
    discoloration, 24, 90, 141, 159
    conditions
        Jue yin cutaneous meridian, 141
        Shao yang cutaneous meridian, 138
        Shao yin cutaneous meridian, 141
        significance, 8, 66
        Tai yang cutaneous meridian, 138
        Tai yin cutaneous meridian, 140
        type T body, 70, 71
        Yang ming cutaneous meridian, 138
    definition, 6
    dermis, 7
    epidermis, 6–7
    functions, 6, 43–44, 48, 137
    meridians, 122; *see also* Cutaneous meridians
        Jue yin, 141
        Shao yang, 139
        Shao yin, 141
        Tai yang, 139
        Tai yin, 140
        Yang ming, 139
    natural antibiotic peptide, 160f
    nourishment, 124–125
    peripheral nervous system damage, 29
    subcutaneous fat, 8–10
    swellings, 4
    TCM and, 8
    thermoregulation and, 7–8
    thyroid gland and, 137
    ulcer, 144
Sleep
    arousal response, 32
    bath and, 150
    disorders, 29, 99, 102

176 • Index

habit, 18, 152–153
    patterns, 20, 156
Sleep apnea, 102
Small intestine, 18, 19, 19f, 47, 51
Smell sensitivity, 63
Smoking, 32
SNS, *see* Sympathetic nervous system (SNS)
Social media networks, 1
Soles, 7, 114, 124
Soleus muscle, 55, 109, 111, 132
Sound sensitivity, 63
Sour taste, 42
Spider veins, 112, 134
Spinalis muscle, 111, 133
Spine, 94, 104, 114
Spleen
    emotions and, 33
    functions in TCM, 14–16
        autonomic nervous system (ANS), 14–15
        dampness, 15
        diaphragm and congestion in abdominal
           cavity, 16
        extremities and muscle, 15–16
        transportation and transformation, 15
    in meridian clock cycle, 19, 19f
    middle Jiao, 18
    taste and, 42
    Zang organs, 51
Splenius capitis muscle, 127, 128
Standing, 100, 112
Staphylococcus sp, 161
Static skin disorder, 62
Sterling, Peter, 36
Sternocleidomastoid (SCM) muscle, 111, 130, 131,
    134
Sternum, 102, 131
Steroid hormones, 33
Stomach, 19, 19f, 44, 51, 153
Stomach Qi, 15
Stress, 7, 8, 11, 15, 32, 42
Stress hyperglycemia, 49
Stress-induced autoimmune disorder, 62
Stress management, 18
Stretch marks (striae), 24, 27, 28
Structure versus function, 50–51
Subcutaneous fat, 8–10, 23–34, 25
Subcutaneous needle, 29
Subdermal tissues, 27
Sublingual glands, 31
Submandibular glands, 31
Subscapularis muscle, 93, 127
Sulfuric acid, 46
Sun dynasty, 159
Superficial blood-letting technique, 145
Supraspinatus, 128

Sway back, *see* Type M2 body
Sweat glands, 7, 8, 29, 41, 43, 160f
Sweating, 7–8, 41, 132
Sweet taste, 42
Sympathetic nervous system (SNS), 3, 6, 15, 54, 83

T

Tai yang meridian, 19, 138–139, 138f
Tai yin meridian, 19, 140, 140f
T cells, 160f
TCM, *see* Traditional Chinese medicine (TCM)
Temporalis muscle, 128, 133
Temporomandibular joint (TMJ), 30–32, 75
Temporomandibular joint disorders (TMD), 31, 94,
    127
Tendinomuscular (muscle) meridians, 122
Tendonitis, 62, 94
Tendons; *see also* Joint pain
    Achilles tendon, 4, 109, 111
    exercise, 49, 50
    nourishment, 124–125
    overweight and obese, 29
    significance, 112
    type M2 body, 101
Tension headache, 62, 66–67
Tensor fascia latae muscle, 27, 101, 133
Teres major muscle, 93, 102
Teres minor muscle, 127
Thenar muscles, 129
Thermoregulation, 7–8, 43, 44
Thirst, 40, 41, 42, 89, 139
Thoracic cavity, 17
Thoracic kyphosis, 102
Thoracic outlet syndrome, 94
Thoracolumbar fascia, 102
Three foot yang meridians, 132–134
    clinical syndrome, 132
    foot Shao yang gallbladder meridian flow, 133,
        133f
    foot Tai yang urinary bladder meridian flow,
        132–133, 132f
    foot Yang ming stomach meridian flow, 133–134,
        134f
Three foot yin meridians, 134–136
    clinical syndrome, 134
    foot Jue yin liver meridian flow, 135, 135f
    foot Shao yin kidney meridian flow, 135–136,
        136f
    foot Tai yin spleen muscle meridian flow,
        134–135, 135f
Three hand yang meridians, 127–128
    clinical syndrome, 127
    hand Shao yang san jiao (triple burner) meridian
        flow, 127–128, 128f

Index • 177

hand Tai yang small intestine meridian flow, 127, 127f

hand Yang ming large intestine meridian flow, 128, 128f

Three hand yin meridians, 128–132
 clinical syndrome, 128–129
 hand Jue yin pericardium muscle meridian flow, 129–130, 129f
 hand Shao yin heart meridian flow, 130, 130f
 hand Tai yin lung muscle meridian flow, 129, 129f
 hand Yin muscle meridian reference, 130–132

Thyroid gland, skin and, 137
Thyroid hormones, 82
Tibialis anterior muscle, 109, 134, 142
Tingling, 29, 92
TMD, *see* Temporomandibular joint disorders (TMD)
TMJ, *see* Temporomandibular joint (TMJ)
Toe pain, 108, 112
Tongue observation, 159
Torticollis, 94
Traditional Chinese medicine (TCM)
 blood flow, 63
 burn treatment, 28
 Chinese medicine, balance, and homeostasis, 36–37
 diagnostic techniques, 159
 healthy condition, 14
 life cycles, 37–39
 biological rhythms, 38
 kidney and kidney essence, 38–39
 overview, 37–38
 meridian system, 13–20
 Asian and Western medicine, 20
 body cavities and body fluids, 16–18
 circadian rhythms and the meridian clock, 19–20
 essentials, 13–14
 healthy habits and circadian rhythm, 18
 obesity, 14
 sleep and wakefulness, 20
 spleen, 14–16
 skin and, 8
 taste and organ disharmony, 42
 Wu Xing, 37
Transformation, 17
Transverse abdominis muscle, 102, 131, 131f, 134
Trapezius muscle, 93, 101, 128, 131, 133
Trauma, 29, 41
Treatise on Cold Damage Disorders (220 A.D.), 44
Treatise on Cold Injury (220 A.D.), 44
Treatment methods, 143–154
 clinical setting, 143–149
 acupressure, 148–149
 cardiac pulmonary resuscitation (CPR), 148
 cupping, 144–145

gastrointestinal resuscitation (GIR), 147–148
 hyperthermal methods, 146–147
 moxa oil and gua sha, 145–146
 muscle meridian acupuncture technique, 143–144
 home setting, 149–154
 diet and nutrition, 152–153
 half-body bath, 149–150
 muscle meridian stretching, 150–152
 personal planning, 153–154
 type M1 body, 94
 type M2 body, 105–106
 type M3 body, 115
 type P body, 68
 type S body, 85
 type T body, 76
receivers
 adhesion-related disorders (ARD), 25–26
 body reshaping and successful health regimens, 22–23
 bruxism, 32
 caesarian section (C-section), 24–25
 cellulite, 28
 depression and anxiety, 32–33
 emotional expression by the body, 29–30
 functional gastrointestinal disorders (FGID), 26–27
 major scars, 27–28
 medications history complications, 33
 obesity, 33–34
 peripheral neuropathies, 28–29
 postchildbirth complications, 24
 subcutaneous fat, 23–24
 temporomandibular joint (TMJ), 30–32
 weight loss or diet life versus your life, 21–22
 three foot yang meridians, 132–134
 three foot yin meridians, 134–136
 three hand yang meridians, 127–128
 three hand yin meridians, 128–132
 type M2 body, 104–105
 type M3 body, 114–115
 type P body, 67–68
 type S body, 84–85
 type T body, 75–76
Triceps brachii muscle, 23, 127
Triple burner, *see* San Jiao (Triple Burner)
True Qi, 15
Type M1 body, 89–98
 associated disorders, 94
 body posture and face conditions, 159
 case study, 94–98
 clinical syndrome, 90
 criteria, 61
 gastrointestinal resuscitation (GIR) and moxa treatment, 156

178 • Index

home therapy and caution, 94
illustrative examples, 61f, 90f
mechanism, 90–92, 91f
moxa oil and gua sha, 156
muscle connection and function, 93
neck wrinkle, 91f
pain, 92–93
postural characteristics, 93–94
quick tips, 89
related condition, 89–90
type P body and, 63, 67, 90, 93
yang, 90, 92, 139f
yin, 90, 92, 93
Type M1 yang, 90, 92, 127, 139f
Type M1 yin, 90, 92, 93, 128
Type M2 body, 98–107
adhesions and, 26
associated disorders, 104
body posture and face conditions, 159
case study, 106–107
clinical syndrome, 99–100
criteria, 61
gastrointestinal resuscitation (GIR) and moxa
treatment, 156
home care and precautions, 105–106
illustrative examples, 61f, 98f
mechanism, 100–101, 101f, 103f
muscle connections and functions, 101–103
pain, 103–104
pillow stretching, 151
postural characteristics, 104
quick tips, 98–99
three foot yan meridians and, 132
treatment, 104–105
type P body and, 67
Type M3 body, 107–119
associated disorders, 114
blood circulation, 113
body posture and face conditions, 159
case study, 116–119
clinical syndrome, 108–110
criteria, 61
gastrointestinal resuscitation (GIR) and moxa
treatment, 156
home therapy and precautions, 115
illustrative examples, 61f
mechanism, 110–111, 110f
moxa oil and gua sha, 156
muscle sequential connection and function,
111–112
neck wrinkle, 91f
pain, 113–114
postural characteristics, 114
quick tips, 107–108
related condition, 108

temporomandibular disorders (TMD), 32
treatment, 114–115
type P body and, 67
Type P body, 62–70
acupressure and, 149
associated disorders, 67
body posture and face conditions, 162
case study, 68–70
clinical syndrome, 63–65
body trunk depressed and extremities
pressed, 63–64
body trunk pressed and extremities
depressed, 63
skin tension—muscle weak, 64
skin weak—muscle tension, 64–65
criteria, 61
dampness pattern, 18
definition, 65, 65f
eating and, 152
home therapy and caution, 68
illustrative example, 61f, 62f
mechanism, 65–66, 65f
muscle meridian acupuncture technique, 155, 156
neck wrinkle, 91f
pain, 66–67, 75
postural characteristics, 67
quick tips, 62
related conditions, 62–63
treatment, 67–68
type M1 body and, 63, 67, 90, 93
Type S body, 78–87
associated disorders, 84
case study, 85–87
clinical syndrome, 79–82
Chong and Yin Wei Type, 79–80, 80f
Dai and Yang Wei Type, 80, 80f
Du and Yang Qiao Type, 81–82, 81f
Ren and Yin Qiao Type, 80, 81f
criteria, 61
definition, 79
extraordinary channels and, 39
home therapy and caution, 85
illustrative examples, 61f, 78f
mechanism, 82–83
moxa soap and, 150
pain, 83–84
postural characteristics, 84
quick tips, 78
related conditions, 78–79
treatment, 84–85
type P pattern and, 64
Type T body, 70–78
acupressure and, 149
associated disorders, 75
body posture and face conditions, 162

case study, 76–78
clinical syndrome, 71–72
criteria, 61
dampness pattern, 18
definition, 71, 71f
home therapy and caution, 76
illustrative examples, 61f, 70f
mechanism, 72–74
moxa soap and, 150
pain, 74–75
postural characteristics, 75
quick tips, 70
related conditions, 70–71
three foot meridians, 132
treatment, 75–76
type P pattern and, 64

U

Ulcerative colitis, 147
Ulcers, 112, 145
Ultradian rhythms, 38
Underweight, 49
Upper Jiao, 17
Urea, 46
Uric acid, 84
Urinary bladder, 19, 19f, 25, 51
Urination, 29, 108, 134
U.S. National Health and Nutrition Examination Survey (NHANES), 33

V

Vacuity and repletion identification, 40
Vacuity patterns, 40
Valgus knee shape, 103
Varicose veins, 73, 114, 134
Vasoconstriction, 43, 44, 65, 149
Vastus medialis muscle, 135
Vein problems, 134
Venous insufficiency, 73, 114, 137, 149
Visceral fat, 8–9
Vitamin D, 47, 48, 137

W

Wakefulness, 20
Walking, 16, 26, 49
Water, 41
Water intake, 41–43
Weakness

allergic reaction, 157
hypocalcemia, 47
lower back, 102
neuropathies, 28, 141
respiratory acidosis, 46
three foot yang meridians, 124
type T body, 71
Weight gain, 24, 33, 71, 73, 132
Weight loss, 12, 21–22, 108
Wei level, 39
Wei Qi, 56
Western medicine, 16, 20; see also Traditional Chinese medicine (TCM)
Wet-cupping therapy, 145
Wind bi, 83
Wind-heat pattern, 17
Winged scapular (scapular alata), 94, 127
World Health Organization (WHO), 33, 98
Worry, 33
Wound healing, 27
Wrinkles, 8, 9, 162
Wrist flexors, 142
Wu Xing, 37

X

Xue level, 39

Y

Yang and yin identification, 40
Yang channels, 52
Yang heel meridian, 54–55, 55f
Yang linking meridian, 55–57, 56f
Yang ming meridian, 19, 139, 139f
Yin and yang, 36, 40
Yin dynasty, 36, 52
Ying level, 39
Yin heel meridian, 54–55, 55f
Yin linking meridian, 55–57, 56f

Z

Zang organs, 51
Zeitgebers, 38
Zhen, Li Shi, 51
Zhong Jing, Zhang (张仲景), 39, 44
Zhou dynasty, 36
Zygomaticus muscle, 128
Zzim jil bang (heat stone room sauna), 147

An environmentally friendly book printed and bound in England by www.printondemand-worldwide.com

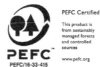

This book is made of chain-of-custody materials; FSC materials for the cover and PEFC materials for the text pages.